SUCCESS!

in Understanding
EKGs

Brenda M. Beasley
BS, RN, EMT-Paramedic

Michael C. West
MS, RN, EMT-Paramedic

Brady
is an imprint of

Pearson

Boston   Columbus   Indianapolis   New York   San Francisco   Upper Saddle River
Amsterdam   Cape Town   Dubai   London   Madrid   Milan   Munich   Paris   Montreal   Toronto
Delhi   Mexico City   Sao Paulo   Sydney   Hong Kong   Seoul   Singapore   Taipei   Tokyo

Library of Congress Cataloging-in-Publication Data

Beasley, Brenda M.
  Success! in understanding EKGs / Brenda M. Beasley, Michael C. West.
    p. cm.
  ISBN-13: 978-0-13-515283-6
  ISBN-10: 0-13-515283-6
  1. Electrocardiography.   I. West, Mike, (Date)–II. Title.
  [DNLM: 1. Electrocardiography—Problems and Exercises. WG 18.2 B368s 2010]
  RC683.5.E5B373 2010
  616.1'207547—dc22   2009007707

Publisher: Julie Levin Alexander	**Production Liaison:** Faye Gemmellaro
Publisher's Assistant: Regina Bruno	**Production Editor:** Ravi Bhatt, Aptara®, Inc.
Editor-in-Chief: Marlene McHugh Pratt	**Manufacturing Manager:** Ilene Sanford
Senior Managing Editor for Development: Lois Berlowitz	**Manufacturing Buyer:** Pat Brown
Associate Editor: Monica Moosang	**Creative Director:** Jayne Conte
Director of Marketing: Karen Allman	**Cover Design:** Solid State Graphics
Executive Marketing Manager: Katrin Beacom	**Interior Design:** Janice Bielawa
Marketing Specialist: Michael Sirinides	**Composition:** Aptara®, Inc.
Marketing Assistant: Judy Noh	**Printer/Binder:** Edwards Brothers
Managing Editor for Production: Patrick Walsh	**Cover Printer:** Lehigh-Phoenix Color/Hagerstown

Brady
is an imprint of

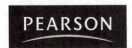

www.bradybooks.com

10 9 8 7 6 5 4 3 2 1
ISBN 13: 978-0-13-515283-6
ISBN 10:   0-13-515283-6

Dedication

This book is dedicated to three amazing people who are, and have always been, my very dearest and most loyal friends,
my sisters,
Hilda (Messer) Camp, Jackie (Messer) Cottle, & Rhonda (Messer) Rogers
With sincere gratitude for their enduring belief in,
and support of me, both personally and professionally.
I love you all dearly!
And to the memory of my parents, Mr. and Mrs. Jack Messer,
My true heroes!

BMB

I would like to dedicate this book to my amazing family who have supported me over the last several years in my many trips away to write this book, my wife Ginger and my children, Christopher and Nikki, as well as my FIVE grandchildren!! Thank you for all of your support.

Also, I would like to add a special thank you to my parents, Barbara West and the late Elmer West, who is and was my inspiration.

MCW

Contents

Foreword

During the course of my career, I have found myself in the position of both student and teacher perhaps more often than most. I have seen health care as a volunteer EMT, a paid Paramedic, a registered nurse, a continuing education instructor, a full-time Paramedic instructor, and now as an Emergency Physician. Of all the academic subjects I have encountered, there is one area of study that seems to be particularly daunting to students of all kinds: EKG interpretation. In addition, unlike subjects such as anatomy, EKG interpretation frequently directly dictates patient care under stressful and emergency conditions. A solid foundation in EKG interpretation is the basis of many health care fields.

It is said that anyone can write a book, and, indeed, there are many texts on EKG interpretation. The mark of a good educator is the ability to synthesize complex information and distill it into a simple, easy-to-understand format. That mark has been met in this text. This book is a continuation in a fine series of EKG texts that take the reader from novice to master of basic principles in an easy-to-follow format. The workbook format is perfect for EKG interpretation because practice is just as vital as understanding the concepts. The text is appropriate for the learner of any level: EMT/Paramedic, nurse, EKG technician, midlevel practitioner, and even medical student. In fact, my peers in medical school frequently lamented that there was no satisfactory EKG text in the medical library, and I would point them toward the Beasley and West books as a foundational text.

I have been blessed to work side by side with both of the authors over the years. Ms. Beasley is a hero in the world of EMS. She is a pioneer, a prolific writer, a consummate educator, a champion for the role of EMS, an example of impeccable integrity, an industrious colleague, and—most importantly—a dear and unyielding friend. Without her vision, wisdom, and selflessness, I would not be the person I am today. Her example and dedication has impacted more lives than she will ever realize.

Mr. West brings more than 20 year of experience in EMS, as well as nursing, to this project. I have been privileged to work alongside (as well as under) Mr. West in countless venues. He is a terrific leader and tireless educator.

It is with great pleasure and excitement that I introduce this fine work into the body of medical literature. This book, like others by these gifted authors, will undoubtedly become a benchmark in EKG texts, shaping young minds from various health care fields, and serving the ultimate goal of all of us in the health professions, eliminating the suffering and premature deaths of our fellow men and women.

Eric Greenfield, DO, NREMT-P
Resident Physician, Emergency Medicine
Medical College of Georgia
Augusta, Georgia

Preface

This workbook consists of chapters that are designed to provide you, the user, with a comprehensive review of ECG strips, as well as a brief overview of core knowledge information relative to ECG interpretation. We trust that you will find the workbook inclusive, user-friendly, and comprehensive in its approach to the review of various ECG strips.

The workbook serves as a stand-alone review book and is appropriate for use in many disciplines, including in-hospital as well as prehospital care. This workbook is intended for the health care provider market at both the basic and advanced levels of understanding and reviewing ECGs. The categories of students who will benefit from this text include prehospital care providers, medical students, cardiac care monitor techs, ACLS candidates, nursing professionals, physician assistants, respiratory therapy students, and cardiac technology students.

It is our hope that you will find this workbook to be beneficial to your knowledge, comprehension, and review of basic ECG interpretation. Your suggestions and comments are always welcome.

Brenda M. Beasley, RN, BS, EMT-Paramedic
E-mail address: bjm18@aol.com

Michael C. West, RN, MS, EMT-Paramedic
E-mail address: MikeWe@alhnet.org

Reviewers

John L. Beckman, AA, BS,
 FF/EMT-P Instructor
Addison Fire Protection District
Addison, IL
Technology Center of DuPage
Fire Science Instructor
Addison, IL

Steven V. Day, NREMTP Instructor
Baxter Regional Medical Center
Education Coordinator
Mountain Home, AR

Russell E. Engle, Jr., BS, NREMTP
Assistant Director, EMS Training
Star Technical Institute
Philadelphia, PA

Phil Ester, EMS Instructor
High Plains Technology Center
Woodward, OK

Brian Hendrickson, EMT-P
Associate Professor/Clinical
 Coordinator
Victor Valley College
Paramedic Academy
Victorville, CA

Colin R. James, NREMT-P
San Francisco Paramedic
 Association
San Francisco, CA

Scott C. Jones, MBA, EMTP
Director, Paramedic Academy
Chairperson, Allied Health
Victorville, CA

Steven M. Kincaid, NR/CCEMTP,
 EMD
Durham County EMS
Durham, NC

Sean Kivlehan, NREMT-P EMS
 Instructor
St. Vincent's Hospital-Manhattan
New York, NY

Lawrence Linder, Hillsborough
 Community College EMS
Tampa, FL

Mike McEvoy, EMS Coordinator
Saratoga County, NY

Pat Patterson, EMT-P, Curriculum
Instructor of EMS
Wake Technical Community
College
Raleigh, NC

John N. Schupra, BSc, CCEMTP,
EMS I/C
Critical Care Program Faculty
Kellogg Community College
Battle Creek, MI

Scott R. Snyder, BS, NREMT-P
Primary EMT Instructor
San Francisco Paramedic
Association
San Francisco, CA

Matthew J. Tatum, NREMTP
Henry County Department of Public
Safety
Martinsville, VA

Carl Voskamp, EMS Program
Coordinator
The Victoria College
Victoria, TX

About the Authors

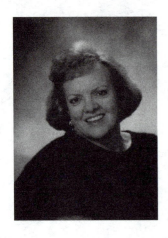

Brenda Messer Beasley is a paramedic and a registered nurse. She earned her bachelor's degree, as well as additional postgraduate studies, from the University of Alabama. Following graduation from nursing school at the University of Alabama, Ms. Beasley was employed as a nurse in the Emergency Department of University Hospital in Birmingham. She remained in emergency nursing for the next 10 years, with a 2-year hiatus when she became certified as a critical care neurosurgical nurse and worked in an NICU at Carraway Medical Center.

Ms. Beasley was working as an ER nurse in 1978 when she was asked to teach a basic EMT course. With a great deal of reticence yet strong encouragement from the chief of staff at the local hospital, she concurred. She immediately developed a passion for quality EMS education, and the rest is history. For the next 30 years, she served as an EMS educator in the state of Alabama, and in 2001 was named Department Chair of Allied Health at Calhoun Community College in Decatur, Alabama. She held that position until her retirement in 2007.

Ms. Beasley has been an affiliate faculty member of the American Heart Association's Emergency Cardiac Care Program for the past 25 years. Other professional activities include BTLS affiliate faculty and board of directors of the National Association of EMS Educators, and she serves on the medical advisory board of 24-7ems.

In 1999, Ms. Beasley published her first book on EKG interpretation, and she has since authored other texts for Brady/Pearson Health Science. She resides in Wedowee, Alabama, where she serves as vice-chair of the local hospital board. Ms. Beasley is actively involved in the First United Methodist Church of Wedowee.

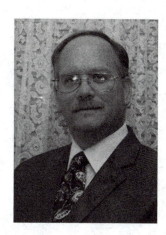

Michael C. West is an EMT-Paramedic and a registered nurse. He earned his associate's degrees in EMS, Nursing, and Police Science from Calhoun Community College. He earned his bachelor's degree from Athens State College and his master's degree from Auburn University at Montgomery. Mr. West was initially employed at Athens Limestone Hospital as an EMT-Basic. His Intermediate training and Paramedic training were done at the University of Alabama in Huntsville program. He went part-time at Athens Limestone Hospital EMS to work at the TVA Brownsferry Nuclear Plant for 2 years as a public safety officer providing fire/police/EMS services. In 1980, Athens Limestone Hospital offered him the position of director of emergency services for the hospital-based EMS system. He returned there full-time and is presently serving in that position.

After getting his RN, Mr. West worked PRN at Huntsville Hospital's emergency department and has moved to PRN status with Huntsville Hospital's Critical Care Transport Services as a transport nurse. Mr. West was an adjunct instructor and taught EMT-Intermediate and EMT-Paramedic classes at the University of Alabama in Huntsville, as well as with the University of Alabama in Birmingham when the program was taken over by them. When the EMS program was moved to Calhoun Community College, Mr. West started as an adjunct instructor at that institution.

At Calhoun Community College, Mr. West and Ms. Beasley got together and decided that a 12-lead book was needed at the basic level to introduce students to the art of reading 12-lead EKGs, and they collaborated to co-author *12-Lead EKGs: A Practical Approach* for Brady.

Mr. West resides in Athens, Alabama, where he also serves as the coroner for Limestone County. He is active in the American Heart Association as an instructor in ACLS, PALS, and BLS courses, as well as a PEPP instructor. He is also an instructor in TNCC with the Emergency Nurses Association.

Refresher Features: The Heart and Its Functions

Refresher Features:

- The heart is located in the mediastinum. See Figure 1-1.
- The heart lies in front of the spinal column, behind the sternum and between the lungs. See Figure 1-1.
- Due to its size and shape, roughly two-thirds of the heart is located to the left of the midline. See Figure 1-1.
- The apex (bottom) of the heart lies just above the diaphragm. See Figure 1-1.
- The (top) base of the heart lies at approximately the level of the third rib. See Figure 1-2.
- The shape of the heart is "conelike" in appearance. See Figure 1-2.
- It is appropriate to visualize the heart as approximately the size of the owner's closed fist. See Figure 1-2.
- There are four hollow chambers in the normal heart. See Figure 1-3.
- On each side of the heart, there is an upper chamber, which is referred to as the atrium {atria—plural}, and a lower chamber known as the ventricle. See Figure 1-3.
- Surrounding the heart is a closed, two-layered sac referred to as the pericardium, also known as the pericardial sac. The pericardial sac contains a small amount of fluid (10–30 mL), which acts to prevent friction between surfaces as the heart contracts. See Figure 1-4.

Figure 1-1 Location of the heart within the chest

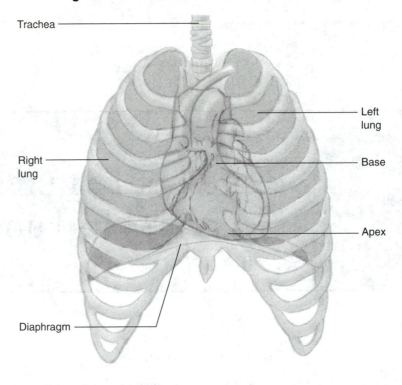

Figure 1-2 Position and orientation of the heart

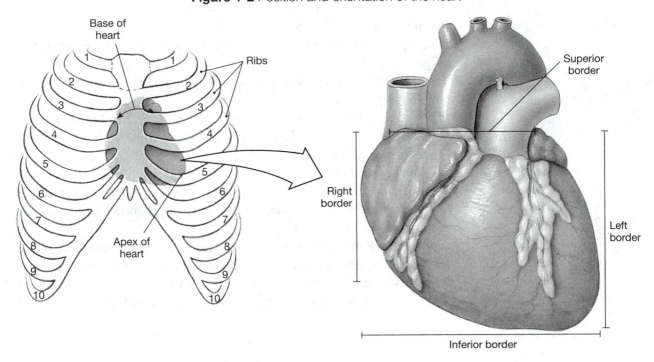

Figure 1-3 Chambers of the heart

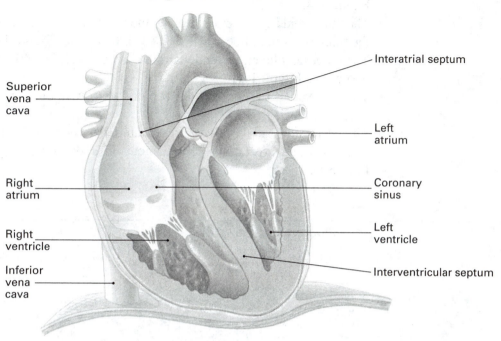

Interatrial septum

Superior vena cava

Left atrium

Right atrium

Coronary sinus

Right ventricle

Left ventricle

Inferior vena cava

Interventricular septum

Figure 1-4 Layers of the heart

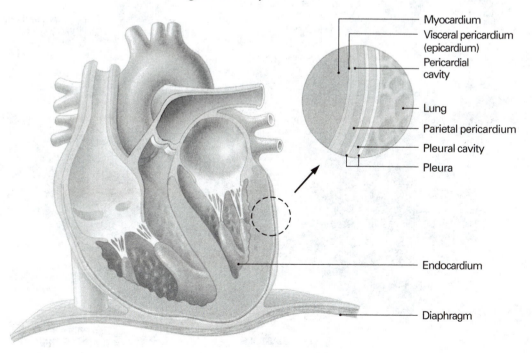

Myocardium

Visceral pericardium (epicardium)

Pericardial cavity

Lung

Parietal pericardium

Pleural cavity

Pleura

Endocardium

Diaphragm

- The epicardium accounts for the smooth outer surface of the heart. See Figure 1-4.
- The thick, middle, muscular layer of the heart is the myocardium and is the thickest of the three layers of the heart wall. See Figure 1-4.
- The innermost layer, the endocardium, is comprised of thin connective tissue. See Figure 1-4.
- The four valves of the heart allow blood to flow in only one direction. See Figure 1-5.
- The atrioventricular valves are located between the atria and the ventricles and are known as the bicuspid and tricuspid valves. See Figure 1-5.

Figure 1-5 Valves of the heart

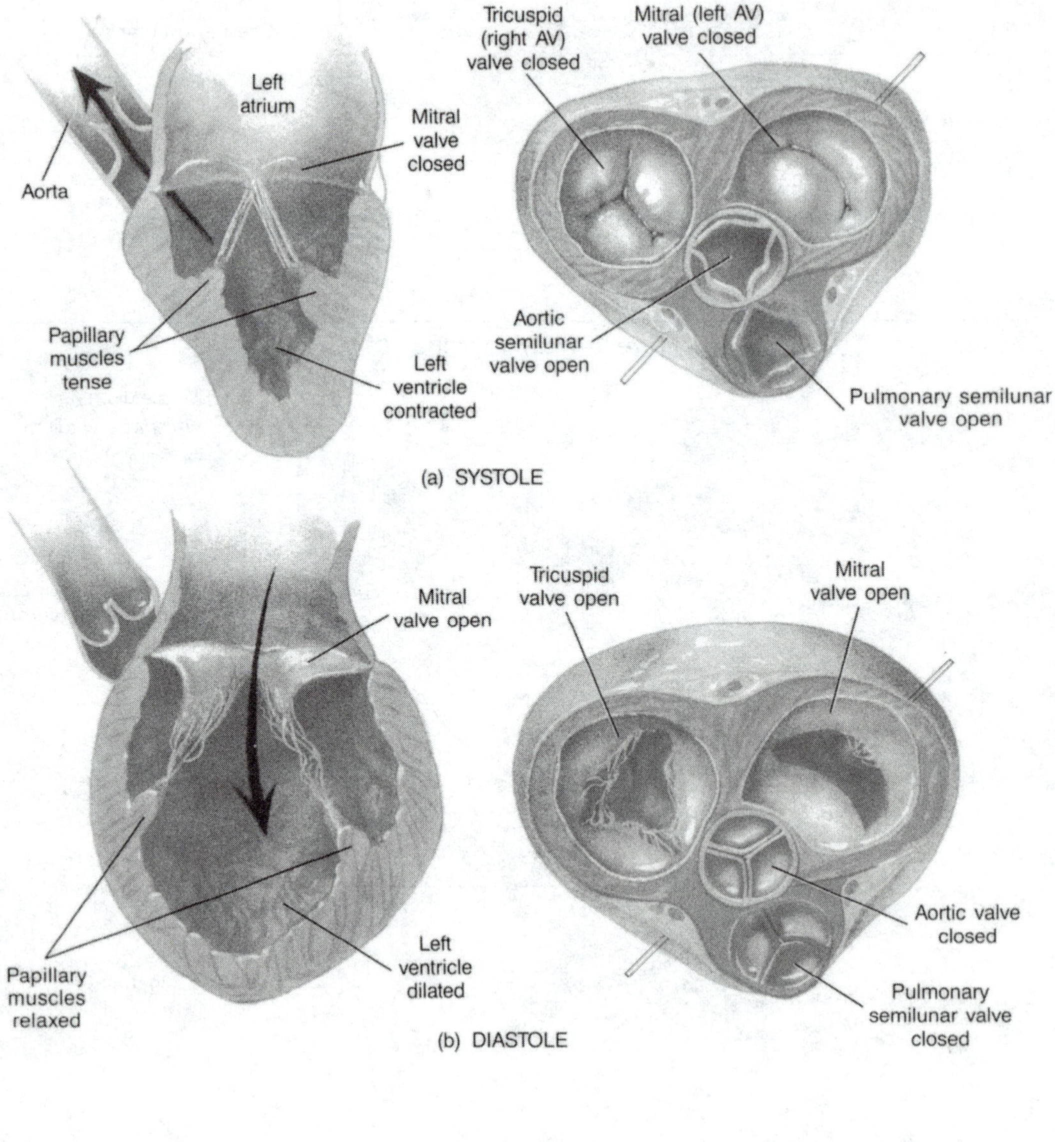

(a) SYSTOLE

(b) DIASTOLE

Figure 1-6 Arterial wall layers

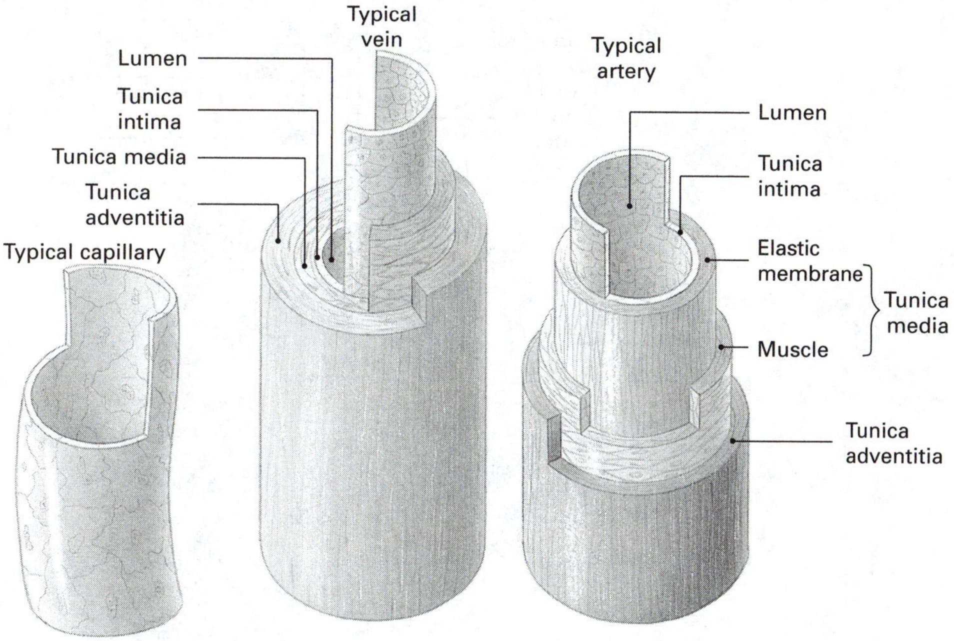

- The AV valves allow blood to flow from the atria into the ventricles and prevent backflow into the atria. See Figure 1-5.
- The semilunar valves serve to prevent the backflow of blood into the ventricles. See Figure 1-5.
- Each semilunar valve contains three semilunar (or moon-shaped) cusps. The semilunar valves are the pulmonic and aortic valves. See Figure 1-5.
- Arteries are relatively thick walled and muscular in makeup. See Figure 1-6.
- Arteries function under high pressure in order to convey blood from the heart out to the rest of the body. See Figure 1-6.
- Veins are defined as "blood vessels that carry blood back to the heart." See Figure 1-7.
- Veins operate under low pressure, are relatively thin walled, and contain one-way valves. See Figure 1-7.
- Capillaries are tiny blood vessels whose walls are the thinnest of all blood vessels. See Figure 1-8.
- Capillaries allow for the exchange of oxygen, nutrients, and waste products between the blood and body tissues and are viewed as "connectors" between arteries and veins. See Figure 1-8.
- The right atrium functions, in part, to receive unoxygenated blood from the head, neck, trunk, and extremities. See Figure 1-9.

Figure 1-7 Coronary circulation

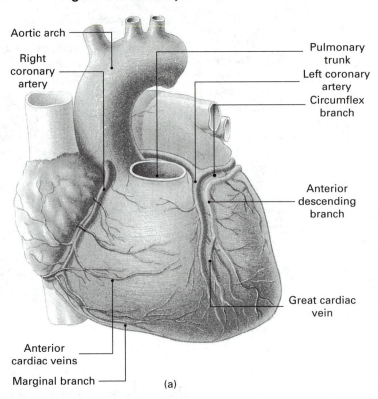

Aortic arch

Right coronary artery

Pulmonary trunk

Left coronary artery

Circumflex branch

Anterior descending branch

Great cardiac vein

Anterior cardiac veins

Marginal branch

(a)

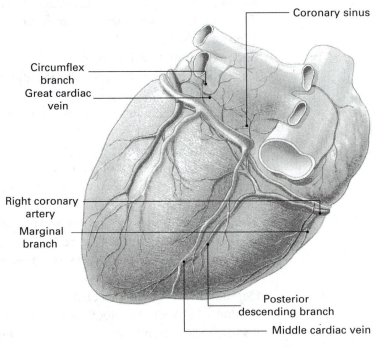

Coronary sinus

Circumflex branch

Great cardiac vein

Right coronary artery

Marginal branch

Posterior descending branch

Middle cardiac vein

(b)

Figure 1-8 Organization of capillary beds

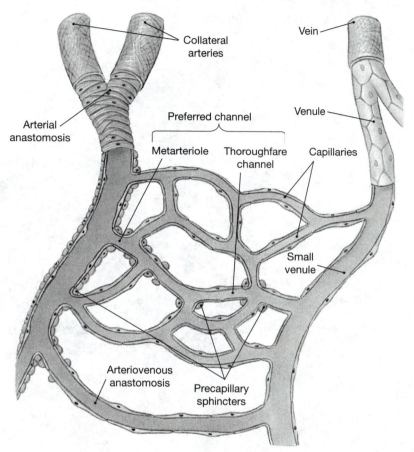

- The right ventricle receives blood from the right atrium and pumps to the pulmonary system. See Figure 1-9.
- The left atrium receives oxygenated blood from the pulmonary system. See Figure 1-9.
- The left ventricle receives this oxygenated blood from the left atrium and pumps it to the head and body systems. See Figure 1-9.
- The cardiac cycle represents the time from initiation of ventricular contraction to initiation of the next ventricular contraction. See Figure 1-10.
- Systole (ventricular systole) is consistent with simultaneous contraction of the ventricles. Remember that atrial systole (contraction of the atrium) occurs first. See Figure 1-10.
- Diastole is synonymous with atrial and ventricular relaxation. See Figure 1-10.
- Stroke volume refers to the volume of blood pumped out of one ventricle of the heart in a single beat or contraction.

Figure 1-9 Blood flow through the heart

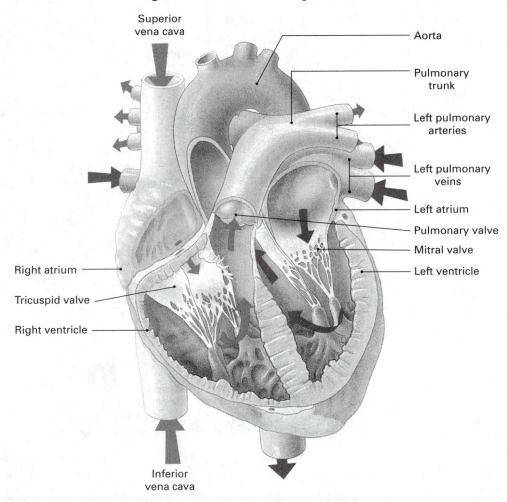

Superior
vena cava

Aorta

Pulmonary
trunk

Left pulmonary
arteries

Left pulmonary
veins

Left atrium

Pulmonary valve

Mitral valve

Left ventricle

Right atrium

Tricuspid valve

Right ventricle

Inferior
vena cava

Cardiac output [CO] = Stroke volume (SV) × heart rate (HR)

- Stroke volume is estimated at 70 cc per beat.
- Cardiac output is the amount of blood pumped by the left ventricle in 1 min.
- Also called end-diastolic volume, preload is the pressure in the ventricles at the end of diastole.
- Afterload is the resistance against which the heart must pump.
- When the volume of blood in the ventricles is increased, stretching the ventricular myocardial fibers causes a more forceful contraction. This concept is known as Starling's law of the heart.

Figure 1-10 Cardiac cycle

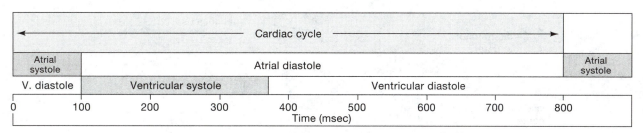

Atrial systole	Atrial diastole	Atrial systole
V. diastole	Ventricular systole	Ventricular diastole

Cardiac cycle

0   100   200   300   400   500   600   700   800

Time (msec)

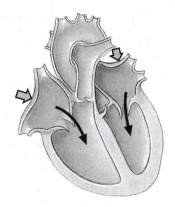

Atrial systole
(a)

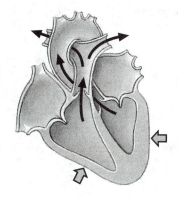

Ventricular systole
(b)

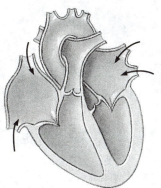

Early ventricular diastole
(c)

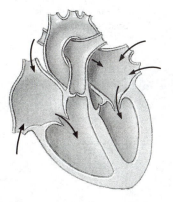

Late ventricular diastole
(d)

Figure 1-11 Nervous control of the heart

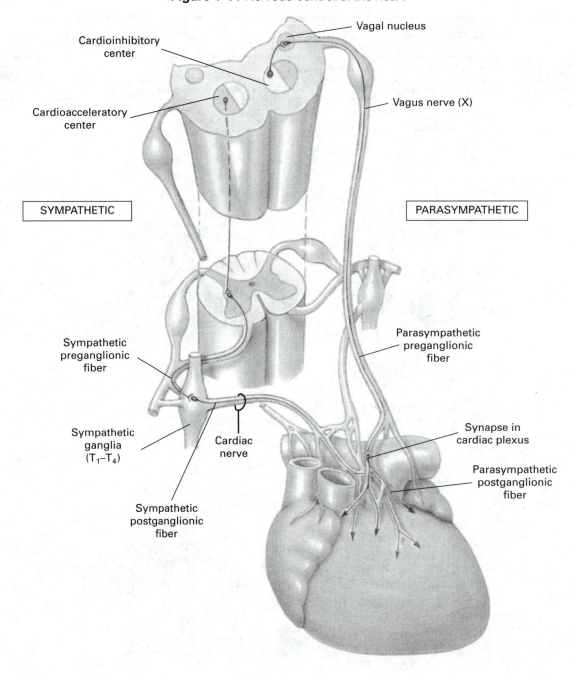

- The autonomic nervous system regulates functions of the body that are involuntary or are not under conscious control. Heart rate and blood pressure are regulated by this component of the nervous system. See Figure 1-11.

- There are two major divisions of the autonomic nervous system: the sympathetic nervous system and the parasympathetic nervous system. See Figure 1-11.
- The sympathetic nervous system is responsible for preparation of the body for physical activity ("fight or flight"). This system is responsible for increasing heart rate and the strength of cardiac contractions. See Figure 1-11.
- The parasympathetic nervous system regulates the calmer ("rest and digest") functions of our existence. This system is responsible for decreasing heart rate. See Figure 1-11.

Electrophysiology and the ECG

Refresher Features:

- The myocardial working cells are responsible for generating the physical contraction of the heart muscle. See Figure 2-1.
- The specialized pacemaker cells are responsible for controlling the rate and rhythm of the heart by coordinating regular depolarization and are found in the electrical conduction system of the heart. See Figure 2-1.
- *Automaticity* is the ability of cardiac pacemaker cells to spontaneously generate their own electrical impulses without external (or nervous) stimulation.
- *Excitability* is the ability of cardiac cells to respond to an electrical stimulus. This characteristic is shared by all cardiac cells and is also referred to as irritability.
- *Conductivity* is the ability of cardiac cells to receive an electrical stimulus and to then transmit the stimulus to other cardiac cells.
- *Contractility* is the ability of cardiac cells to shorten and cause cardiac muscle contraction in response to an electrical stimulus.
- Potassium plays a role in cardiac depolarization and has a major function in repolarization.
- Sodium plays a vital part in depolarization of the myocardium.
- Calcium renders an important function in myocardial depolarization and myocardial contraction.

Figure 2-1 Cardiac muscle cell

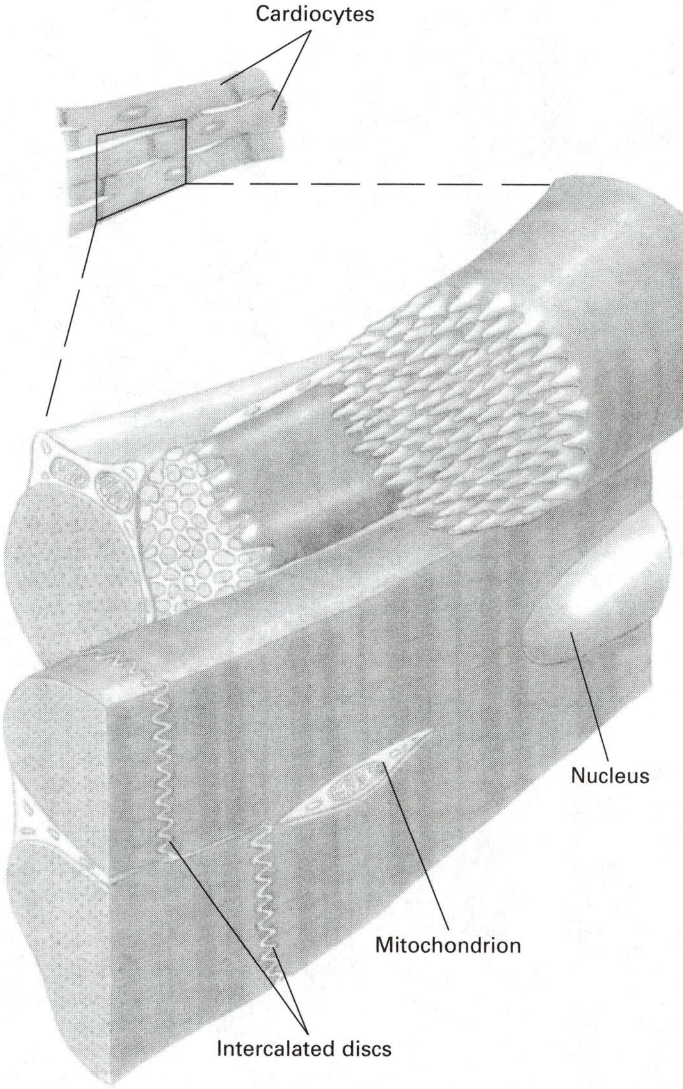

Cardiocytes

Nucleus

Mitochondrion

Intercalated discs

- When the cardiac cell is at rest, the potassium ion concentration is greater inside the cell than outside, and the sodium ion concentration is greater outside the cell than inside.
- By means of an active mechanism of transport called the sodium-potassium exchange pump, potassium and sodium ions are moved in and out of the cell through the cell membrane.
- *Depolarization* is an electrical occurrence resulting in myocardial contraction and involving the movement of ions across cardiac cell membranes, which results in positive polarity inside the cell membrane. See Figure 2-2.

Figure 2-2 Depolarization and repolarization

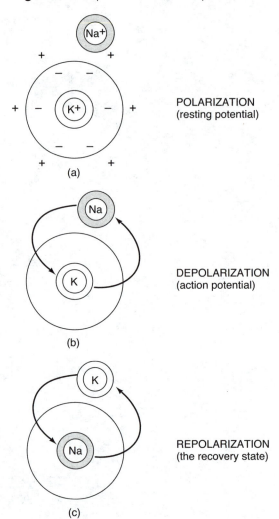

POLARIZATION
(resting potential)

(a)

DEPOLARIZATION
(action potential)

(b)

REPOLARIZATION
(the recovery state)

(c)

- Repolarization is a process whereby the depolarized cell is polarized, so the positive charges are again on the outside, with negative charges on the inside of the cell—a return to the resting state.
- During the majority of the process of repolarization, the cardiac cell is unable to respond to a new electrical stimulus; the cardiac cell cannot spontaneously depolarize and is referred to as the *absolute refractory period*. (This begins with the first deflection of the QRS complex and ends near the upslope of the T wave.) See Figure 2-3.
- The *relative refractory period* is the period when repolarization is almost complete and the cardiac cell can be stimulated to contract prematurely if the stimulus is much stronger than normal (downslope of the T wave).

Figure 2-3 Refractory periods

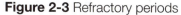

Absolute refractory period   Relative refractory period

Figure 2-4 Bipolar lead placement

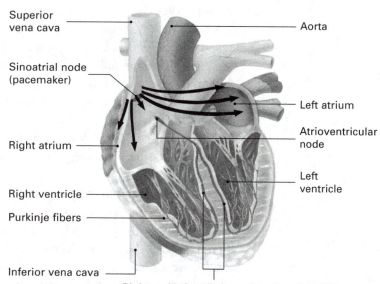

Superior vena cava

Sinoatrial node (pacemaker)

Right atrium

Right ventricle

Purkinje fibers

Inferior vena cava

Aorta

Left atrium

Atrioventricular node

Left ventricle

Right and left branches of the bundle of His

- On the ECG strip, the relative refractory period corresponds with the downslope of the T wave and is termed the vulnerable period of repolarization.
- The SA (or sinoatrial) node is located in the upper posterior portion of the right atrial wall of the heart and is the pacemaker of the heart, with an intrinsic firing rate of 60 to 100 bpm.
- The SA node generates impulses that travel throughout the muscle fibers of both atria, resulting in depolarization.
- Three internodal tracts, or pathways, receive the electrical impulse as it exits the SA node. See Figure 2-4.
- The internodal pathways distribute the electrical impulse throughout the atria and transmit the impulse from the SA node to the AV node.
- The AV (or atrioventricular) node is located on the floor of the right atrium just above the tricuspid valve, with an intrinsic firing rate of 40 to 60 bpm, which is slower than the SA node. It will become the pacemaker if the SA node fails.

- The AV junction is where the internodal pathways leading from the SA node join the bundle of His.
- The bundle of His leads out of the AV node.
- The bundle of His is referred to as the common bundle.
- The bundle of His divides into two main branches at the top of the interventricular septum, the right bundle branch and the left bundle branch.
- The primary function of the bundle branches is to conduct electrical activity from the bundle of His down to the Purkinje network.
- The Purkinje fibers are a network of small conduction fibers that spread throughout the ventricles.
- The Purkinje fibers carry electrical impulses directly to ventricular muscle cells. They have an intrinsic firing rate of 20 to 40 bpm, which is slower than both the SA and AV nodes. They will assume pacemaker responsibilities if both the SA and AV nodes fail.
- An *electrode* is an adhesive pad that contains conductive gel and is designed to be attached to the patient's skin.
- Electrodes are connected to the monitor or ECG machine by wires called *leads*.
- Leads I, II, and III are known as bipolar leads (standard limb leads), which means that these leads have one positive electrode and one negative electrode.
- The left arm lead may be placed at a location between the left shoulder and wrist for diagnostic 12-lead or for monitoring the left upper chest. Be sure to stay away from bony prominences. See Figure 2-5.
- The right lead should be placed between the right shoulder and wrist for diagnostic 12-lead or for monitoring the right upper chest. Again, be sure to stay away from bony prominences.
- The left leg lead should be placed between the left hip and ankle for diagnostic 12-lead or for monitoring the upper left abdomen.

Figure 2-5 ECG placement

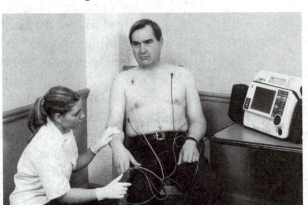

Figure 2-6 Standard limb leads

Limb lead placement

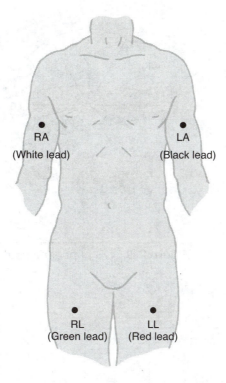

Figure 2-7 Augmented leads

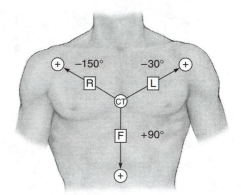

- The right leg lead is placed between the right hip and ankle for diagnostic 12-lead or for monitoring the right upper abdomen. This is sometimes utilized as an additional ground lead. See Figure 2-6.

Note: The following five points are included informationally for those readers who are interested in lead placement for 12-lead ECGs:

- With the augmented limb leads, the current flows from the heart outward to the extremities and is amplified by the ECG machine; hence the name augmented or extended from the heart.
- Augmented leads (aVR, aVF, aVL) are referred to as unipolar (having only one true pole) leads and utilize the 4 limb leads that are the second set of 3 leads with the 12-lead ECG. This adds a fourth ground lead as the base. See Figure 2-7.
- The precordial (chest) leads are unipolar and comprise the last 6 leads on the 12-lead ECG.
- The precordial (chest) leads look at the heart via the horizontal (or transverse) plane.
- The precordial (chest) leads are also called precordial or V (vector) leads. Proper placement of the V leads is critically important to the correct interpretation of the 12-lead ECG strip. See Figure 2-8.

Figure 2-8 12-lead ECG

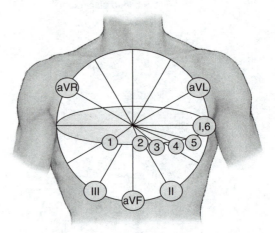

Figure 2-9 ECG paper and markings

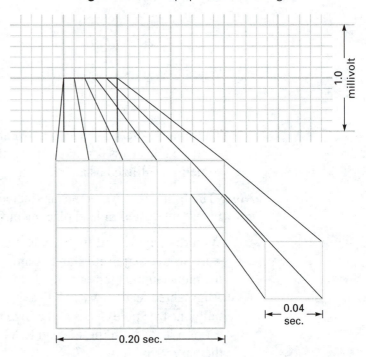

- Electrocardiographic paper is arranged as a series of horizontal and vertical lines printed on graph paper and provides a printed record of cardiac electrical activity. See Figure 2-9.
- ECG paper leaves the machine at a constant speed of 25 mm/s for a standard 3 lead or 12 lead.
- Time is measured on the horizontal line, while amplitude or voltage is measured on the vertical line.

Figure 2-10 The P wave

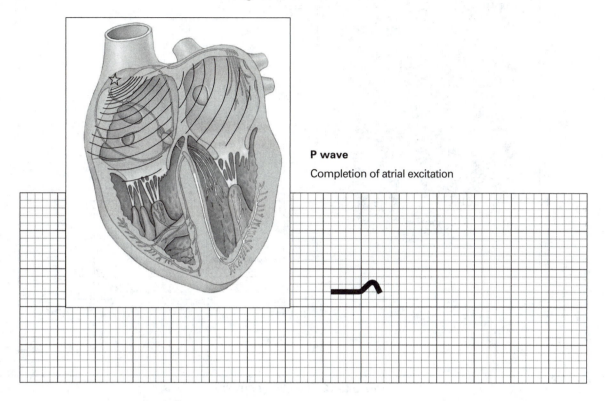

P wave
Completion of atrial excitation

- The vertical axis reflects millivolts (2 large squares = 1 mV and 1 mV = 10 mm).
- ECG graph paper is divided into small squares, each of which is 1 mm in height and width and represents a time interval of 0.04 seconds.
- Darker lines further divide the paper every fifth square, both vertically and horizontally.
- The squares on the ECG paper represent the measurement of the length of time required for the electrical impulse to traverse a specific part of the heart.
- A wave or waveform recorded on an ECG strip refers to movement away from the baseline (isoelectric line).
- Waveforms are represented as a positive deflection (above the isoelectric line) or as a negative deflection (below the isoelectric line).
- The P wave represents depolarization of both the left and right atria. See Figure 2-10.
- The PR interval represents the time interval necessary for the impulse to travel from the SA node, through the internodal pathways in the atria, and downward to the ventricles. See Figure 2-11.
- The QRS complex represents the conduction of the electrical impulse from the bundle of His throughout the ventricular muscle, or ventricular depolarization. See Figure 2-12.

Figure 2-11 The P-R interval

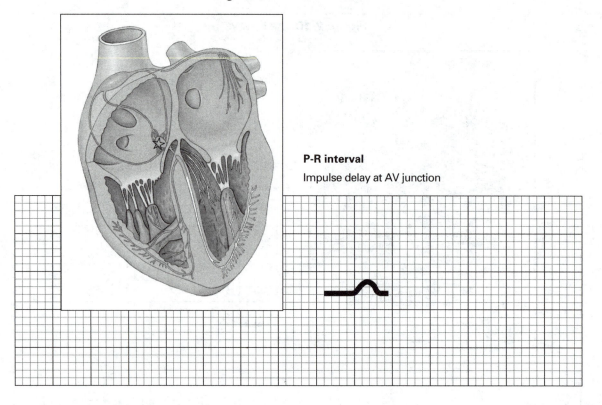

P-R interval

Impulse delay at AV junction

Figure 2-12 The QRS complex

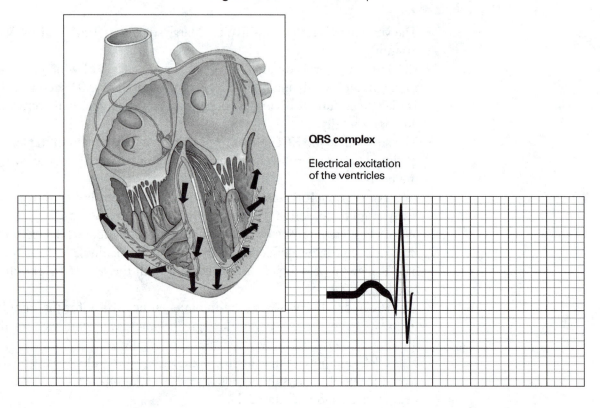

QRS complex

Electrical excitation
of the ventricles

Figure 2-13 The J point

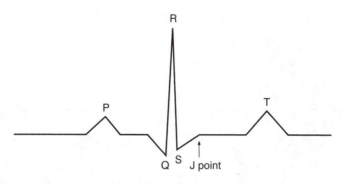

Figure 2-14 The T wave

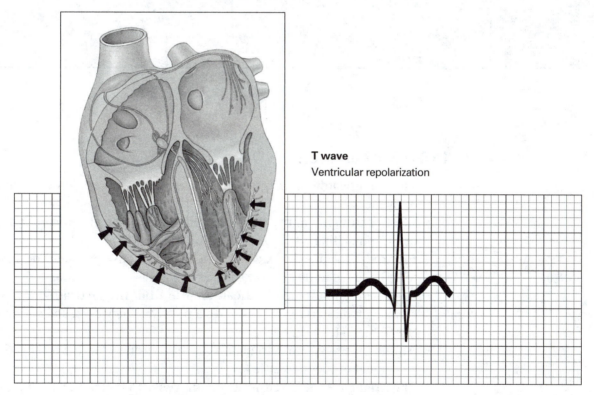

T wave
Ventricular repolarization

- The J point is the point at which the QRS complex meets the ST segment. See Figure 2-13.
- The ST segment is the interval during which the ventricles are depolarized; ventricular repolarization begins and is called the ST segment.
- The T wave represents ventricular repolarization. See Figure 2-14.

Review of Three-Lead ECGs

Refresher Features:

- The Electrocardiogram: graphic representation of the electrical activity of the heart.
- Electrocardiograph: the machine used to record the electrocardiogram, or ECG machine.
- Electrode: an adhesive pad that contains conductive gel and is designed to be attached to the patient's skin.
- Lead wires: relay the electrical impulse from the myocardium to the cardiac monitor; 3 leads must have a positive, a negative, and a ground. See Table 3-1.
- An imaginary inverted triangle is formed around the heart by proper placement of the bipolar leads.
- This triangle is referred to as Einthoven's triangle. See Figure 3-1. The top of the triangle is formed by Lead I, the right side of the triangle is formed by Lead II, and the left side of the triangle is formed by Lead III.
- Each lead represents a different look at, or view of, the heart.
- For the sake of consistency, chest Lead II will be used throughout this textbook, except where otherwise designated.
- ECG waveforms are recorded on an ECG strip and refer to movement away from the baseline or isoelectric line in a positive or negative deflection.

Table 3-1 Bipolar lead placement

Lead	Positive Electrode	Negative Electrode
I	Left arm	Right arm
II	Left leg	Right arm
III	Left leg	Left arm

Figure 3-1 Einthoven's triangle

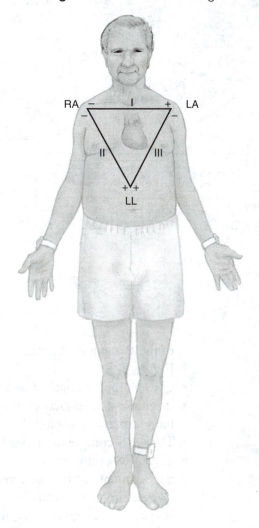

- The first positive deflection is referred to as the P wave and is the impulse generated by the SA node; this impulse travels throughout the myocardium and represents the depolarization of the atria. See Figure 3-2.
- PR Interval: Time impulse travels from SA node through internodal pathways in atria toward ventricles; the time interval from the start

Figure 3-2 P wave

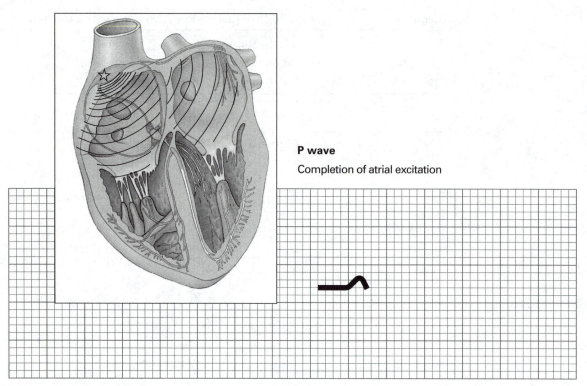

P wave

Completion of atrial excitation

of the P wave to the start of QRS is 0.12–0.20 seconds in length. See Figure 3-3.

- QRS Complex consists of a Q wave, an R wave, and an S wave.
- It represents conduction of the impulse from the bundle of His through the ventricular muscle.
- The QRS complex represents ventricular depolarization.
- The QRS complex measures less than 0.12 seconds. See Figure 3-4.
- ST Segment is the time interval during which the ventricles are depolarized and repolarization of the ventricles begins.
- It starts at the end of the QRS complex and ends at the upswing of the T wave. See Figure 3-5.
- The T wave follows the ST segment and represents ventricular repolarization.
- It is the resting phase of the cardiac cycle.
- One complete cardiac cycle is the P wave, the QRS complex, the ST segment, and the T wave. See Figure 3-6.

Figure 3-3 PR interval

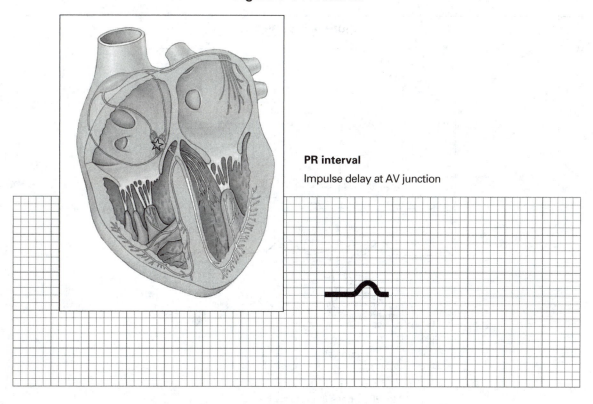

PR interval

Impulse delay at AV junction

Figure 3-4 QRS complex

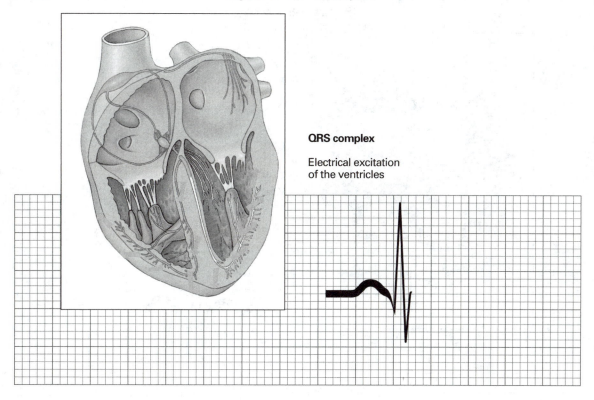

QRS complex

Electrical excitation
of the ventricles

Figure 3-5 ST segment

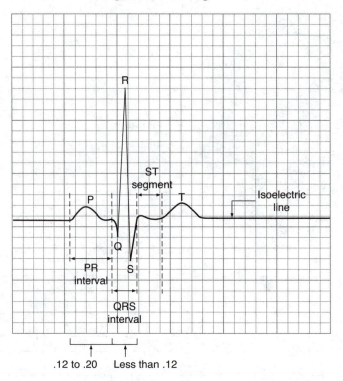

Figure 3-6 T wave

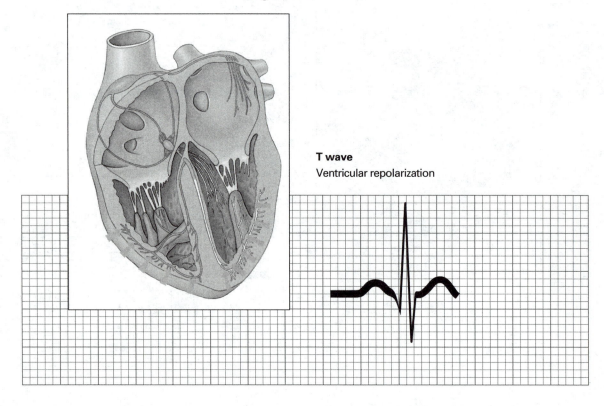

T wave
Ventricular repolarization

Normal Sinus Rhythm: See Table 3-2 and Figure 3-7

Now it is time for you to analyze the rhythm strip in Figure 3-7 and write in your answers to each step of the five-step approach or your preferred method of rhythm strip analysis. The answers are located at the end of this chapter.

Rate: _____

Rhythm: _____

P wave: _____

PR interval: _____

QRS complex: _____

Table 3-2 Normal sinus rhythm

Questions 1–5	Answers
1. What is the rate?	60–100 bpm
2. What is the rhythm?	Atrial rhythm regular; ventricular rhythm
3. Is there a P wave before each QRS?	Yes
Are the P waves upright and uniform?	Yes
4. What is the length of the PR interval?	0.12–0.20 seconds (3–5 small squares)
5. Do all the QRS complexes look alike?	Yes
What is the length of the QRS complexes?	Less than 0.12 seconds (3 small squares)

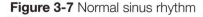

Figure 3-7 Normal sinus rhythm

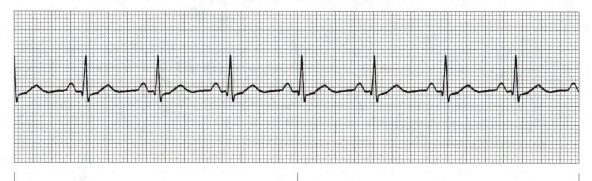

Sinus Bradycardia: See Table 3-3 and Figure 3-8

Now it is time for you to analyze the rhythm strip in Figure 3-8 and write in your answers to each step of the five-step approach. The answers are located at the end of this chapter.

Rate: _____

Rhythm: _____

P wave: _____

PR interval: _____

QRS complex: _____

Table 3-3 Sinus bradycardia rhythm

Questions 1–5	Answers
1. What is the rate?	Less than 60 bpm
2. What is the rhythm?	Atrial rhythm regular; ventricular rhythm regular
3. Is there a P wave before each QRS?	Yes
Are the P waves upright and uniform?	Yes
4. What is the length of the PR interval?	0.12–0.20 seconds (3–5 small squares)
5. Do all the QRS complexes look alike?	Yes
What is the length of the QRS complexes?	Less than 0.12 seconds (3 small squares)

Figure 3-8 Sinus bradycardia rhythm

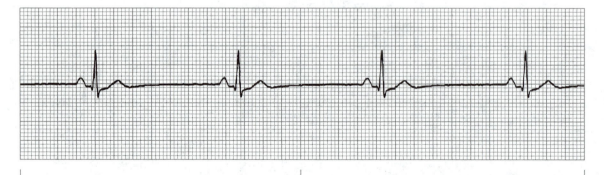

Sinus Tachycardia Rhythm: See Table 3-4 and Figure 3-9

Now it is time for you to analyze the rhythm strip in Figure 3-9 and write in your answers to each step of the five-step approach. The answers are located at the end of this chapter.

Rate: _____

Rhythm: _____

P wave: _____

PR interval: _____

QRS complex: _____

Table 3-4 Sinus tachycardia rhythm

Questions 1–5	Answers
1. What is the rate?	100–160 bpm
2. What is the rhythm?	Atrial rhythm regular; ventricular rhythm regular
3. Is there a P wave before each QRS? Are the P waves upright and uniform?	Yes Yes
4. What is the length of the PR interval?	0.12–0.20 seconds (3–5 small squares)
5. Do all the QRS complexes look alike? What is the length of the QRS complexes?	Yes Less than 0.12 seconds (3 small squares)

Figure 3-9 Sinus tachycardia rhythm

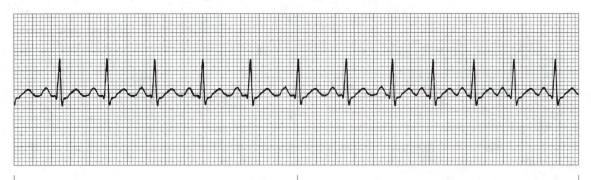

Sinus Dysrhythmia: See Table 3-5 and Figure 3-10

Now it is time for you to analyze the rhythm strip in Figure 3-10 and write in your answers to each step of the five-step approach. The answers are located at the end of this chapter.

Rate: _____

Rhythm: _____

P wave: _____

PR interval: _____

QRS complex: _____

Table 3-5 Sinus dysrhythmia rhythm

Questions 1–5	Answers
1. What is the rate?	60–100 bpm
2. What is the rhythm?	Irregular (variance of more than 0.08 seconds)
3. Is there a P wave before each QRS?	Yes
Are the P waves upright and uniform?	Yes
4. What is the length of the PR interval?	0.12–0.20 seconds (3–5 small squares)
5. Do all the QRS complexes look alike?	Yes
What is the length of the QRS complexes?	Less than 0.12 seconds (3 small squares)

Figure 3-10 Sinus dysrhythmias rhythm

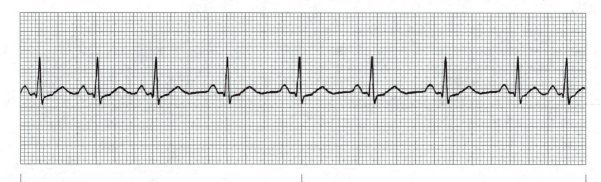

Sinus Arrest Rhythm: See Table 3-6 and Figure 3-11

Now it is time for you to analyze the rhythm strip in Figure 3-11 and write in your answers to each step of the five-step approach. The answers are located at the end of this chapter.

Rate: _____

Rhythm: _____

P wave: _____

PR interval: _____

QRS complex: _____

Table 3-6 Sinus arrest rhythm

Questions 1–5	Answers
1. What is the rate?	Variable, depending on the frequency of sinus arrest
2. What is the rhythm?	Irregular, when sinus arrest is present
3. Is there a P wave before each QRS? Are the P waves upright and uniform?	Yes—if QRS is present Yes—if QRS is present
4. What is the length of the PR interval?	0.12–0.20 seconds (3–5 small squares)
5. Do all the QRS complexes look alike? What is the length of the QRS complexes?	Yes, when present Less than 0.12 seconds (3 small squares)

Figure 3-11 Sinus arrest rhythm

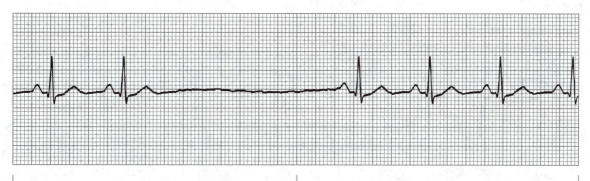

Wandering Atrial Pacemaker: See Table 3-7 and Figure 3-12

Now it is time for you to analyze the rhythm strip in Figure 3-12 and write in your answers to each step of the five-step approach. The answers are located at the end of this chapter.

Rate: _____

Rhythm: _____

P wave: _____

PR interval: _____

QRS complex: _____

Table 3-7 Wandering atrial pacemaker rhythm

Questions 1–5	Answers
1. What is the rate?	Usually 60–100 bpm
2. What is the rhythm?	May be slightly irregular
3. Is there a P wave before each QRS?	Change in shape, size, and location from beat to beat
Are the P waves upright and uniform?	Observation of at least 3 different P waves is required
4. What is the length of the PR interval?	Variable, depending on site shifts
5. Do all the QRS complexes look alike?	Yes
What is the length of the QRS complexes?	Usually less than 0.12 seconds (3 small squares)

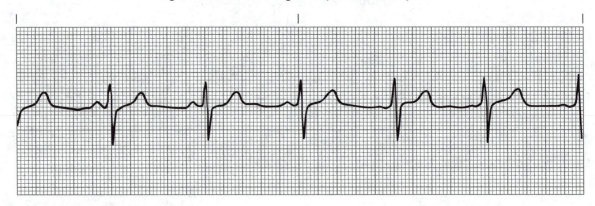

Figure 3-12 Wandering atrial pacemaker rhythm

Multifocal Atrial Tachycardia: See Figure 3-13

Now it is time for you to analyze the rhythm strip in Figure 3-13 and write in your answers to each step of the five-step approach. The answers are located at the end of this chapter.

Rate: _____

Rhythm: _____

P wave: _____

PR interval: _____

QRS complex: _____

Figure 3-13 Multifocal atrial tachycardia

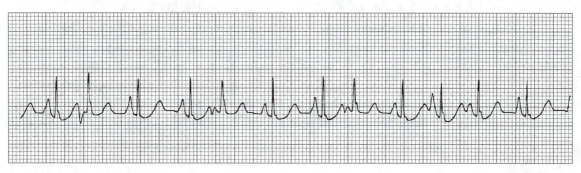

Premature Atrial Complexes: See Table 3-8 and Figure 3-14

Now it is time for you to analyze the rhythm strip in Figure 3-14 and write in your answers to each step of the five-step approach. The answers are located at the end of this chapter.

Rate: _____

Rhythm: _____

P wave: _____

PR interval: _____

QRS complex: _____

Table 3-8 Premature atrial complexes

Questions 1–5	Answers
1. What is the rate?	Usually normal
2. What is the rhythm?	Usually regular, except for PAC
3. Is there a P wave before each QRS? Are the P waves upright and uniform?	Differs in shape, size, and location from normal P waves of rhythm
4. What is the length of the PR interval?	Variable, depending on pacemaker site
5. Do all the QRS complexes look alike? What is the length of the QRS complexes?	Similar to QRS of underlying rhythm; usually less than 0.12 seconds (3 small squares)

Figure 3-14 Premature atrial complexes

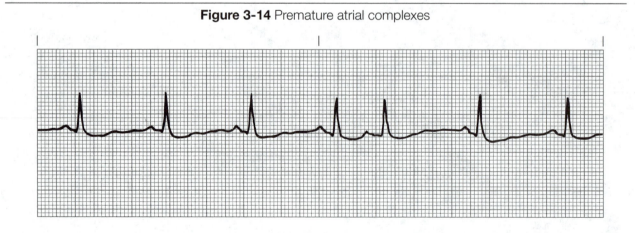

Atrial Flutter Rhythms: See Table 3-9 and Figure 3-15

Now it is time for you to analyze the rhythm strips in Figure 3-15 and write in your answers to each step of the five-step approach. The answers are located at the end of this chapter.

Rhythm A: Rate: _____   *Rhythm B:* Rate: _____

Rhythm: _____   Rhythm: _____

P wave: _____   P wave: _____

PR interval: _____   PR interval: _____

QRS complex: ____   QRS complex: ____

Table 3-9 Atrial flutter

Questions 1–5	Answers
1. What is the rate?	Atrial: 250–300 bpm; ventricular: variable
2. What is the rhythm?	Atrial: regular; ventricular: regular or irregular
3. Is there a P wave before each QRS? Are the P waves upright and uniform?	Normal P waves are absent; replaced by F waves (sawtooth)
4. What is the length of the PR interval?	Not measurable
5. Do all the QRS complexes look alike? What is the length of the QRS complexes?	Usually Less than 0.12 seconds (3 small squares)

Figure 3-15 Atrial flutter

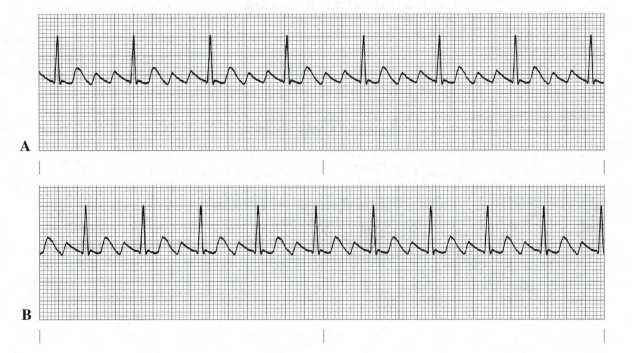

A

B

Atrial Fibrillation Rhythm: See Table 3-10 and Figure 3-16

Now it is time for you to analyze the rhythm strip in Figure 3-16 and write in your answers to each step of the five-step approach. The answers are located at the end of this chapter.

Rate: _____

Rhythm: _____

P wave: _____

PR interval: _____

QRS complex: _____

Table 3-10 Atrial fibrillation

Questions 1–5	Answers
1. What is the rate?	Atrial: 350–400 bpm; ventricular: variable
2. What is the rhythm?	Irregularly irregular
3. Is there a P wave before each QRS? Are the P waves upright and uniform?	Normal P waves are absent; replaced by f waves
4. What is the length of the PR interval?	Not discernable
5. Do all the QRS complexes look alike? What is the length of the QRS complexes?	Yes Usually less than 0.10 seconds

Figure 3-16 Atrial fibrillation

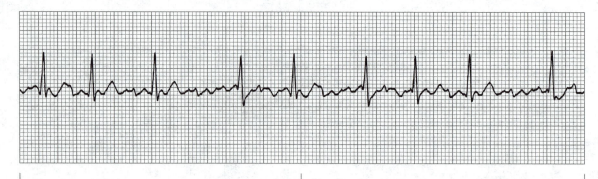

Supraventricular Tachycardia Rhythm: See Table 3-11 and Figure 3-17

Now it is time for you to analyze the rhythm strips in Figure 3-17 and write in your answers to each step of the five-step approach. The answers are located at the end of this chapter.

Rhythm A   Rate: _____   *Rhythm B*   Rate: _____

Rhythm: _____   Rhythm: _____

P wave: _____   P wave: _____

PR interval: _____   PR interval: _____

QRS complex: ____   QRS complex: ____

Table 3-11 Supraventricular tachycardia

Questions 1–5	Answers
1. What is the rate?	Atrial: 150–250 bpm; ventricular: 150–250 bpm
2. What is the rhythm?	Regular
3. Is there a P wave before each QRS? Are the P waves upright and uniform?	Usually not discernible; especially at the high-rate range
4. What is the length of the PR interval?	Usually not discernible
5. Do all the QRS complexes look alike? What is the length of the QRS complexes?	Yes Usually less than 0.10 seconds

Figure 3-17 Supraventricular tachycardia

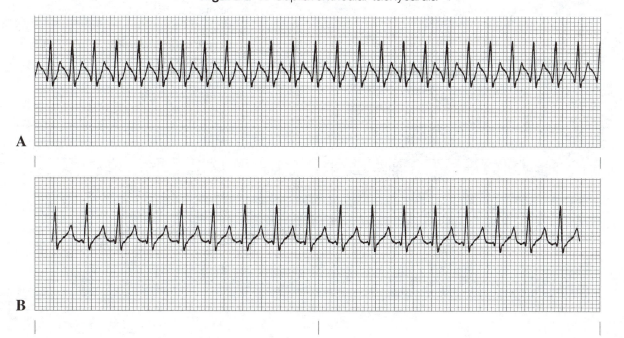

A

B

Premature Junctional Complexes (rhythm): See Table 3-12 and Figure 3-18

Now it is time for you to analyze the rhythm strip in Figure 3-18 and write in your answers to each step of the five-step approach. The answers are located at the end of this chapter.

Rate: _____

Rhythm: _____

P wave: _____

PR interval: _____

QRS complex: _____

Table 3-12 Premature junctional complexes

Questions 1–5	Answers
1. What is the rate?	Rate of underlying rhythm, plus the PJC or PJCs
2. What is the rhythm?	Usually regular, except for premature beat (PJC)
3. Is there a P wave before each QRS? Are the P waves upright and uniform?	Inverted or absent; may appear before or after the QRS
4. What is the length of the PR interval?	Usually less than 0.12 second if P wave precedes QRS; absent if no P wave occurs before the QRS
5. Do all the QRS complexes look alike? What is the length of the QRS complexes?	Yes Less than 0.12 seconds, if no defect in ventricular conduction

Figure 3-18 Premature junctional complexes

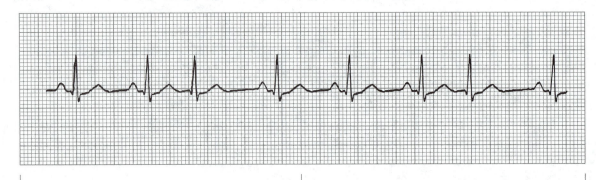

Junctional Escape Rhythms: See Table 3-13 and Figure 3-19

Now it is time for you to analyze the rhythm strip in Figure 3-19 and write in your answers to each step of the five-step approach. The answers are located at the end of this chapter.

Rate: _____

Rhythm: _____

P wave: _____

PR interval: _____

QRS complex: _____

Table 3-13 Junctional escape rhythm

Questions 1–5	Answers
1. What is the rate?	Usually 40–60 bpm
2. What is the rhythm?	Usually regular; irregular if isolated junctional escape beat is present
3. Is there a P wave before each QRS? Are the P waves upright and uniform?	Inverted or absent May appear before or after the QRS
4. What is the length of the PR interval?	Usually less than 0.12 seconds if P wave precedes QRS; absent if no P wave occurs before QRS
5. Do all the QRS complexes look alike? What is the length of the QRS complexes?	Yes Less than 0.12 seconds (3 small squares)

Figure 3-19 Junctional escape rhythm

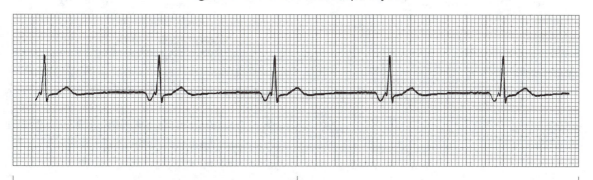

Accelerated Junctional Rhythm: See Table 3-14 and Figure 3-20

Now it is time for you to analyze the rhythm strip in Figure 3-20 and write in your answers to each step of the five-step approach. The answers are located at the end of this chapter.

Rate: _____

Rhythm: _____

P wave: _____

PR interval: _____

QRS complex: _____

Table 3-14 Accelerated junctional rhythm

Questions 1–5	Answers
1. What is the rate?	60–100 bpm
2. What is the rhythm?	Atrial: regular; ventricular: regular
3. Is there a P wave before each QRS? Are the P waves upright and uniform?	Inverted or absent May appear before or after the QRS
4. What is the length of the PR interval?	Usually less than 0.12 seconds if P wave precedes QRS; absent if no P wave occurs before QRS
5. Do all the QRS complexes look alike? What is the length of the QRS complexes?	Yes Less than 0.12 seconds (3 small squares)

Figure 3-20 Accelerated junctional escape rhythm

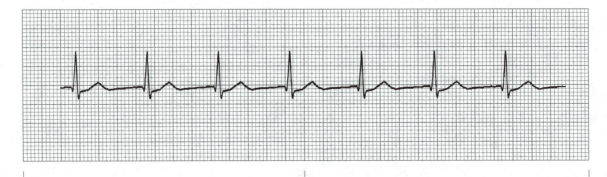

Junctional Tachycardia Rhythm: See Table 3-15 and Figure 3-21

Now it is time for you to analyze the rhythm strip in Figure 3-21 and write in your answers to each step of the five-step approach. The answers are located at the end of this chapter.

Rate: _____

Rhythm: _____

P wave: _____

PR interval: _____

QRS complex: _____

Table 3-15 Junctional tachycardia

Questions 1–5	Answers
1. What is the rate?	100–180 bpm
2. What is the rhythm?	Atrial: regular; ventricular: regular
3. Is there a P wave before each QRS? Are the P waves upright and uniform?	If visible, inverted May appear before or after the QRS
4. What is the length of the PR interval?	Usually less than 0.12 seconds if P wave precedes QRS; absent if no P wave occurs before QRS
5. Do all the QRS complexes look alike? What is the length of the QRS complexes?	Yes Less than 0.12 seconds (3 small squares)

Figure 3-21 Junctional tachycardia

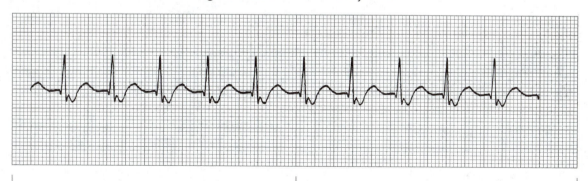

Premature Ventricular Complexes (rhythm): See Table 3-16 and Figure 3-22

Now it is time for you to analyze the rhythm strip in Figure 3-22 and write in your answers to each step of the five-step approach. The answers are located at the end of this chapter.

Rate: _____

Rhythm: _____

P wave: _____

PR interval: _____

QRS complex: _____

Table 3-16 Premature ventricular complexes—unifocal

Questions 1–5	Answers
1. What is the rate?	Dependent on rate of underlying rhythm and number of PVCs
2. What is the rhythm?	Occasionally irregular; regular if interpolated PVC
3. Is there a P wave before each QRS? Are the P waves upright and uniform?	No P waves associated with PVC P waves of underlying rhythm may be present
4. What is the length of the PR interval?	PRI not present with PVCs
5. What do the QRS complexes look like? What is the length of QRS complexes?	Usually wide and bizarre Equal to or greater than 0.12 seconds (3 small squares)

Figure 3-22 Premature ventricular complexes—unifocal

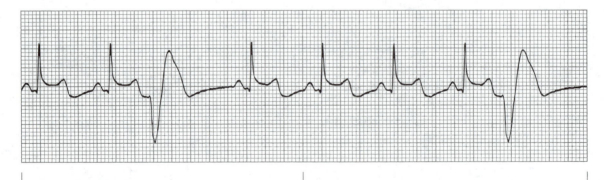

Premature Ventricular Complexes—multifocal: See Figure 3-23

Now it is time for you to analyze the rhythm strip in Figure 3-23 and write in your answers to each step of the five-step approach. The answers are located at the end of this chapter.

Rate: _____

Rhythm: _____

P wave: _____

PR interval: _____

QRS complex: _____

Figure 3-23 Premature ventricular complexes—multifocal

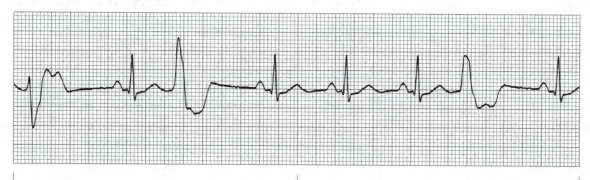

Idioventricular Rhythms: See Table 3-17 and Figure 3-24

Now it is time for you to analyze the rhythm strip in Figure 3-24 and write in your answers to each step of the five-step approach. The answers are located at the end of this chapter.

Rate: _____

Rhythm: _____

P wave: _____

PR interval: _____

QRS complex: _____

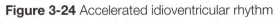

Table 3-17 Accelerated idioventricular rhythm

Questions 1–5	Answers
1. What is the rate?	20–40 bpm or less
2. What is the rhythm?	Atrial rhythm not distinguishable; ventricular rhythm usually regular
3. Is there a P wave before each QRS?	No; none present
4. What is the length of the PR interval?	None
5. Do all the QRS complexes look alike?	Yes; bizarre morphology
What is the length of the QRS complexes?	Greater than 0.12 seconds

Figure 3-24 Accelerated idioventricular rhythm

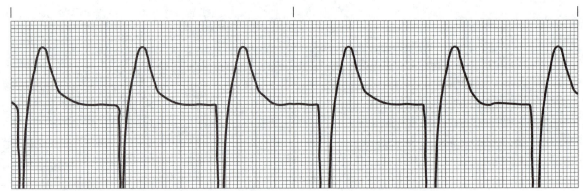

Ventricular Tachycardia Rhythm: See Table 3-18 and Figure 3-25

Now it is time for you to analyze the rhythm strip in Figure 3-25 and write in your answers to each step of the five-step approach. The answers are located at the end of this chapter.

Rate: _____

Rhythm: _____

P wave: _____

PR interval: _____

QRS complex: _____

Table 3-18 Ventricular tachycardia rhythm (fine and coarse)

Questions 1–5	Answers
1. What is the rate?	100–250 bpm
2. What is the rhythm?	Atrial rhythm not distinguishable; ventricular rhythm usually regular
3. Is there a P wave before each QRS?	May be present or absent; not associated with QRS complexes
4. What is the length of the PR interval?	None
5. Do all the QRS complexes look alike?	Yes (except in torsades rhythm); bizarre QRS morphology
What is the length of the QRS complexes?	Greater than 0.12 seconds

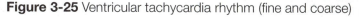

Figure 3-25 Ventricular tachycardia rhythm (fine and coarse)

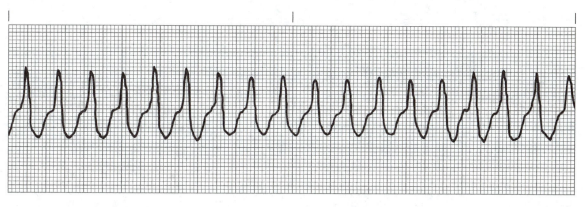

Ventricular Fibrillation Rhythm: See Table 3-19 and Figure 3-26

Now it is time for you to analyze the rhythm strip in Figure 3-26 and write in your answers to each step of the five-step approach. The answers are located at the end of this chapter.

Rate: _____

Rhythm: _____

P wave: _____

PR interval: _____

QRS complex: _____

Table 3-19 Ventricular fibrillation rhythm (fine and coarse)

Questions 1–5	Answers
1. What is the rate?	Rate cannot be discerned
2. What is the rhythm?	Rapid, unorganized; rhythm not distinguishable
3. Is there a P wave before each QRS?	No
4. What is the length of the PR interval?	None present
5. Do all the QRS complexes look alike?	None present
What is the length of the QRS complexes?	None present

Figure 3-26 Ventricular fibrillation rhythm (fine and coarse)

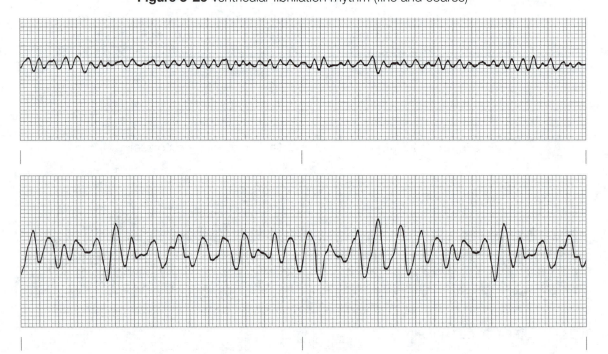

Ventricular Asystole Rhythm: See Table 3-20 and Figure 3-27

Now it is time for you to analyze the rhythm strip in Figure 3-27 and write in your answers to each step of the five-step approach. The answers are located at the end of this chapter.

Rate: _____

Rhythm: _____

P wave: _____

PR interval: _____

QRS complex: _____

Table 3-20 Ventricular asystole

Questions 1–5	Answers
1. What is the rate?	Absent
2. What is the rhythm?	Absent; Rhythm not distinguishable
3. Is there a P wave before each QRS?	No
4. What is the length of the PR interval?	None present
5. Do all the QRS complexes look alike?	None present
What is the length of the QRS complexes?	None present

Figure 3-27 Ventricular asystole

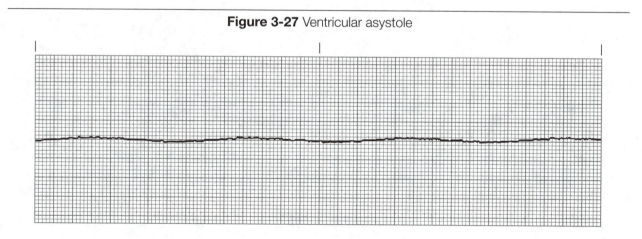

First-Degree AV Block Rhythms: See Table 3-21 and Figure 3-28

Now it is time for you to analyze the rhythm strip in Figure 3-28 and write in your answers to each step of the five-step approach. The answers are located at the end of this chapter.

Rate: _____

Rhythm: _____

P wave: _____

PR interval: _____

QRS complex: _____

Table 3-21 First-degree AV block

Questions 1–5	Answers
1. What is the rate?	Based on the rate of the underlying rhythm
2. What is the rhythm?	Usually regular
3. Is there a P wave before each QRS?	Yes
Are the P waves upright and uniform?	Yes
4. What is the length of the PR interval?	Greater than 0.20 seconds (3–5 small squares)
5. Do all the QRS complexes look alike?	Yes
What is the length of the QRS complexes?	Less than 0.12 seconds(3 small squares)

Figure 3-28 First-degree AV block

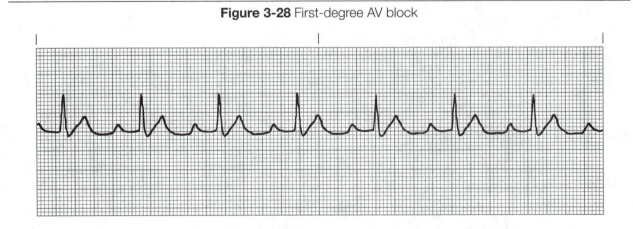

Second-Degree Block (Mobitz Type I): See Table 3-22 and Figure 3-29

Now it is time for you to analyze the rhythm strip in Figure 3-29 and write in your answers to each step of the five-step approach. The answers are located at the end of this chapter.

Rate: _____

Rhythm: _____

P wave: _____

PR interval: _____

QRS complex: _____

Table 3-22 Second-degree AV block (Mobitz type I)

Questions 1–5	Answers
1. What is the rate?	Atrial unaffected; ventricular rate is usually slower than atrial
2. What is the rhythm?	Atrial rhythm regular; ventricular rhythm irregular
3. Is there a P wave before each QRS?	Yes
Are the P waves upright and uniform?	Yes, for conducted beats
4. What is the length of the PR interval?	Progressively prolongs until a QRS is not conducted
5. Do all the QRS complexes look alike?	Yes
What is the length of the QRS complexes?	Less than 0.12 seconds

Figure 3-29 Second-degree AV block (Mobitz type I)

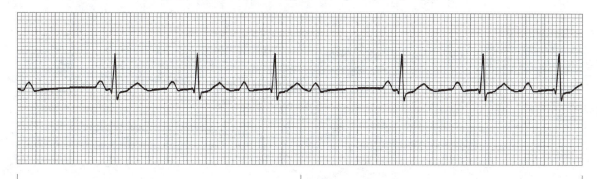

Second-Degree AV Block (Mobitz Type II): See Table 3-23 and Figure 3-30

Now it is time for you to analyze the rhythm strip in Figure 3-30 and write in your answers to each step of the five-step approach. The answers are located at the end of this chapter.

Rate: _____

Rhythm: _____

P wave: _____

PR interval: _____

QRS complex: _____

Table 3-23 Second-degree AV block (Mobitz type II)

Questions 1–5	Answers
1. What is the rate?	Atrial rate regular; ventricular rate may be bradycardic
2. What is the rhythm?	Atrial rhythm regular; ventricular rhythm irregular
3. Is there a P wave before each QRS?	Yes; some P waves are not followed by a QRS complex
Are the P waves upright and uniform?	P waves are usually upright and uniform
4. What is the length of the PR interval?	Constant for conducted beats
5. Do all the QRS complexes look alike? What is the length of the QRS complexes?	Yes; intermittently absent less than or greater than 0.12 seconds

Figure 3-30 Second-degree AV block (Mobitz type II)

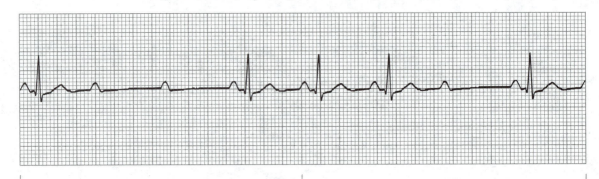

Third-Degree (complete) Heart Block Rhythm: See Table 3-24 and Figure 3-31

Now it is time for you to analyze the rhythm strip in Figure 3-31 and write in your answers to each step of the five-step approach. The answers are located at the end of this chapter.

Rate: _____

Rhythm: _____

P wave: _____

PR interval: _____

QRS complex: _____

Table 3-24 Third-degree (complete) heart block rhythm

Questions 1–5	Answers
1. What is the rate?	Atrial rate usually 60–100 bpm; ventricular rate based on site of escape pacemaker
2. What is the rhythm?	Atrial rhythm regular; ventricular rhythm regular
3. Is there a P wave before each QRS? Are the P waves upright and uniform?	No relationship to QRS complexes Yes
4. What is the length of the PR interval?	Totally variable; no pattern
5. Do all the QRS complexes look alike? What is the length of the QRS complexes?	Yes Based on site of escape pacemaker

Figure 3-31 Third-degree (complete) heart block rhythm

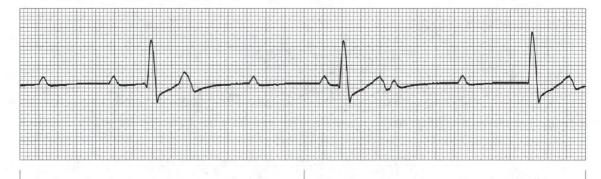

Artificial Pacemaker Rhythm: See Table 3-25 and Figure 3-32

Now it is time for you to analyze the rhythm strip in Figure 3-32 and write in your answers to each step of the five-step approach. The answers are located at the end of this chapter.

Rate: _____

Rhythm: _____

P wave: _____

PR interval: _____

QRS complex: _____

Table 3-25 Artificial pacemaker rhythm

Questions 1–5	Answers
1. What is the rate?	Varies according to preset rate of pacemaker
2. What is the rhythm?	Regular if pacing is fixed; irregular if demand-paced
3. Is there a P wave before each QRS?	May be absent or present, depending on type of artificial pacemaker
Are the P waves upright and uniform?	Pacer spikes may be present; otherwise the P wave will usually be upright and uniform
4. What is the length of the PR interval?	Variable, depending on type of artificial pacemaker
5. Do all the QRS complexes look alike?	Usually; bizarre morphology; presense of spikes
What is the length of the QRS complexes?	Greater than 0.12 seconds

Figure 3-32 Artificial pacemaker rhythm

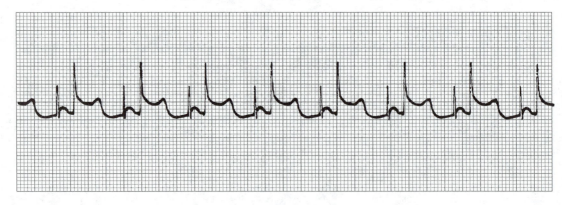

✓answers

Figure 3-7

Rate:	70
Rhythm:	Regular
P wave:	Present and upright
PRI:	0.16
QRS:	0.04

Figure 3-8

Rate:	40
Rhythm:	Regular
P wave:	Present and upright
PRI:	0.16
QRS:	0.04

Figure 3-9

Rate:	120
Rhythm:	Regular
P wave:	Present and upright
PRI:	0.16
QRS:	0.04

Figure 3-10

Rate:	90
Rhythm:	Irregular
P wave:	Present and upright
PRI:	0.16
QRS:	0.04

Figure 3-11

Rate:	60
Rhythm:	Irregular
P wave:	Present and upright
PRI:	0.16
QRS:	0.06

Figure 3-12

Rate:	60
Rhythm:	Regular
P wave:	Present and upright
PRI:	Variable
QRS:	0.08

Figure 3-13

Rate:	120
Rhythm:	Irregular
P wave:	Present and upright
PRI:	Variable
QRS:	0.04

Figure 3-14

Rate:	70
Rhythm:	Irregular
P wave:	Present and upright
PRI:	0.16
QRS:	0.08

Figure 3-15 A

Rate: 80
Rhythm: Regular
P wave: f waves
PRI: Absent
QRS: 0.04

Figure 3-15 B

Rate: 100
Rhythm: Regular
P wave: f waves
PRI: Absent
QRS: 0.04

Figure 3-16

Rate: 90
Rhythm: Irregular
P wave: Absent
PRI: Absent
QRS: 0.04

Figure 3-17 A

Rate: 250
Rhythm: Regular
P wave: Indistinguishable
PRI: Indistinguishable
QRS: 0.04

Figure 3-17 B

Rate: 170
Rhythm: Regular
P wave: Indistinguishable
PRI: Indistinguishable
QRS: 0.06

Figure 3-18

Rate: 80
Rhythm: Irregular
P wave: Present and upright
PRI: 0.16
QRS: 0.04

Figure 3-19

Rate: 50
Rhythm: Regular
P wave: Inverted
PRI: 0.12
QRS: 0.06

Figure 3-20

Rate: 70
Rhythm: Regular
P wave: Absent
PRI: Absent
QRS: 0.06

Figure 3-21

Rate: 100
Rhythm: Regular
P wave: Absent
PRI: Absent
QRS: 0.06

Figure 3-22

Rate: 80
Rhythm: Irregular
P wave: Present and upright
PRI: 0.12
QRS: 0.08

Figure 3-23

Rate: 80
Rhythm: Irregular
P wave: Present and upright
PRI: 0.16
QRS: 0.04

Figure 3-24

Rate: 60
Rhythm: Regular
P wave: Absent
PRI: Absent
QRS: Greater than 0.12

Figure 3-25

Rate: 180
Rhythm: Regular
P wave: Absent
PRI: Absent
QRS: Greater than 0.12

Figure 3-26

Rate: Greater than 200
Rhythm: Irregular
P wave: Absent
PRI: Absent
QRS: Absent

Figure 3-27

Rate: Absent
Rhythm: Absent
P wave: Absent
PRI: Absent
QRS: Absent

Figure 3-28

Rate: 70
Rhythm: Regular
P wave: Present and upright
PRI: 0.26
QRS: 0.08

Figure 3-29

Rate: 60
Rhythm: Irregular
P wave: Present and upright
PRI: Variable
QRS: 0.04

Figure 3-30

Rate: 50
Rhythm: Irregular
P wave: Present and upright
PRI: Variable
QRS: 0.04

Figure 3-31

Rate: 30
Rhythm: Regular
P wave: Present and upright
PRI: Variable
QRS: 0.08

Figure 3-32

Rate: 80
Rhythm: Regular
P wave: Pacer spike
PRI: 0.12
QRS: 0.08

ECG Rhythm Strips and Scenarios

Scenario #1

A 16-year-old male presents with chest pain that started after taking some "pills" at a friend's house. The medication is determined to be a grandparent's Digitalis. The patient's blood pressure is 90/54, heart rate is as shown in the rhythm (Figure 4-1), and respirations are 24 with an oxygen saturation on room air of 95%. You place the patient on the cardiac monitor and it shows the following rhythm.

Utilizing the five-step approach, what is your interpretation of this patient's rhythm strip?

Rate: _____

Rhythm: _____

P wave: _____

PRI: _____

QRS: _____

Scenario #2

A 46-year-old male presents with weakness for a few days, stated he has been taking a blood pressure pill that "a friend" had given to him for the past sev-

Figure 4-1

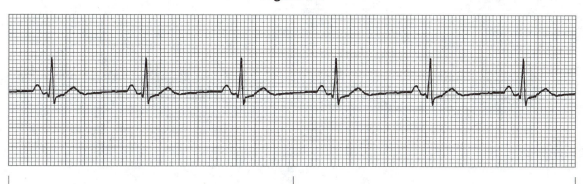

eral days. He states that he checked his blood pressure at a local store on "one of those machines." His blood pressure is 70/40, heart rate is as shown in Figure 4-2, and his oxygen saturation on room air is 95%. You place the patient on the cardiac monitor and it shows the rhythm in Figure 4-2.

Rate: _____

Rhythm: _____

P wave: _____

PRI: _____

QRS: _____

Interpretation of the rhythm strip: _____

Figure 4-2

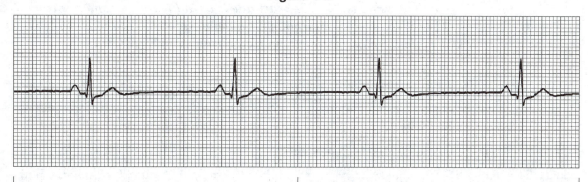

Scenario #3

A 50-year-old male presents with chest pain that started after taking some "cocaine" for the first time. Blood pressure is 170/99; heart rate is as shown

Figure 4-3

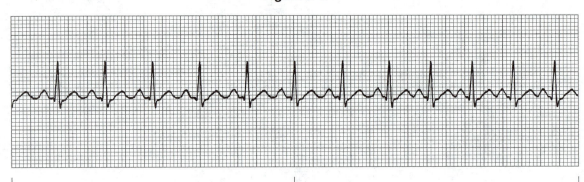

in the rhythm in Figure 4-3, and respirations are 24 with an oxygen saturation on room air of 95%. You place the patient on the cardiac monitor and it shows the rhythm in Figure 4-3.

Rate: _____

Rhythm: _____

P wave: _____

PRI: _____

QRS: _____

Interpretation of the rhythm strip: _____

Scenario #4

A 49-year-old female presents "with a feeling like her heart stops." Her blood pressure is 140/90; heart rate is as in Figure 4-4, and respirations are 22 with an oxygen saturation on room air of 97%. You place the patient on the cardiac monitor and it shows the rhythm in Figure 4-4.

Figure 4-4

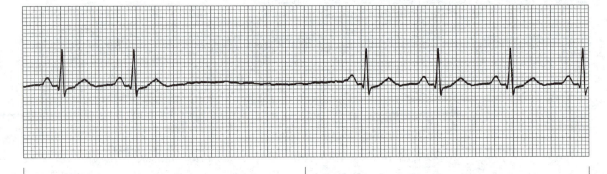

Rate: _____

Rhythm: _____

P wave: _____

PRI: _____

QRS: _____

Interpretation of the rhythm strip: _____

Scenario #5

A 69-year-old female presents "with an irregular heart beat," which began this morning. Blood pressure is 130/88; heart rate is shown in Figure 4-5, and respirations are 22 with an oxygen saturation on room air of 97%. You place the patient on the cardiac monitor, and it shows the rhythm in Figure 4-5.

Rate: _____

Rhythm: _____

P wave: _____

PRI: _____

QRS: _____

Interpretation of the rhythm strip: _____

What medication would most likely be utilized to convert the rhythm?

   a. Atropine
   b. Lidocaine
   c. Cardiozem
   d. Adenosine

Answer: _____

Figure 4-5

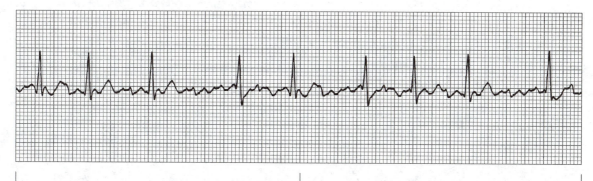

Scenario #6

A 55-year-old female presents and states that she thinks that she has been taking too much of her Lanoxin "and has not been feeling well." Her blood pressure is 107/60; heart rate is as shown in Figure 4-6, and respirations are 24, with an oxygen saturation on room air of 96%. You place the patient on the cardiac monitor, and it shows the rhythm in Figure 4-6.

Rate: _____

Rhythm: _____

P wave: _____

PRI: _____

QRS: _____

Interpretation of the rhythm strip: _____

Figure 4-6

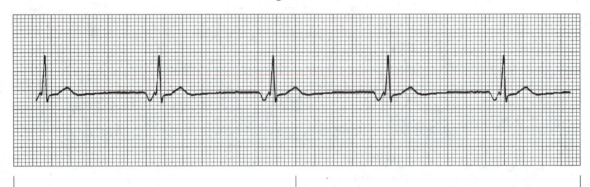

Scenario #7

A 45-year-old male presents and states that he "is having skipped beats in my chest," and it makes him feel funny. His blood pressure is 138/76; heart rate is as shown in Figure 4-7, and respirations are 24 with an oxygen saturation on room air of 96%. You place the patient on the cardiac monitor and it shows the rhythm in Figure 4-7.

Rate: _____

Rhythm: _____

P wave: _____

PRI: _____

QRS: _____

Interpretation of the rhythm strip: _____

Figure 4-7

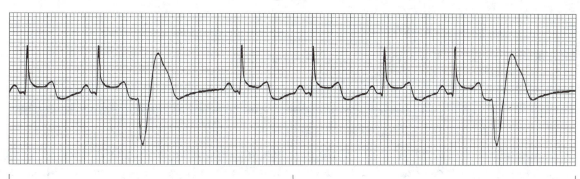

Scenario #8

A 45-year-old male pushes the call button in his hospital room and states that "this feeling of skipped beats in my chest is getting worse." His blood pressure is 122/70; heart rate is as shown in Figure 4-8, and respirations are 24 with an oxygen saturation on room air of 96%. You observe the cardiac monitor and note the following rhythm.

Rate: _____

Rhythm: _____

P wave: _____

PRI: _____

QRS: _____

Interpretation of the rhythm strip: _____

Figure 4-8

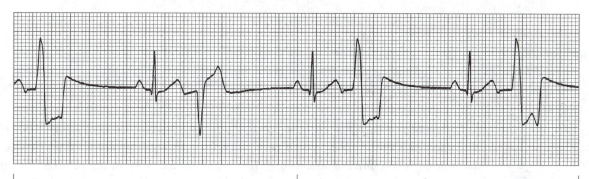

Would you give this patient Lidocaine to stop the ectopic beats?

a. Yes
b. No

Answer: _____

Scenario #9

A 55-year-old male becomes unresponsive sitting in a wheelchair in the cardiac lab after a stress test. He then slumps over. The patient is placed on a stretcher, and he is not breathing and does not have a heart rate. You place the patient on the cardiac monitor, and it shows the rhythm in Figure 4-9.

Rate: _____

Rhythm: _____

P wave: _____

PRI: _____

QRS: _____

Interpretation of the rhythm strip: _____

Figure 4-9

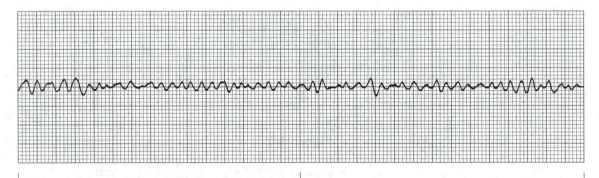

Scenario #10

Mr. Smith was found unresponsive, slumped over in the waiting room of a doctor's office. The patient was placed on a stretcher and was not breathing and did not have a heart rate. You place the patient on the cardiac monitor, and it shows a ventricular fibrillation rhythm. The patient is defibrillated with the appropriate joules and the rhythm shown in Figure 4-10 is noted on the cardiac monitor after 2 min of CPR postshock.

Rate: _____

Rhythm: _____

P wave: _____

PRI: _____

QRS: _____

Interpretation of the rhythm strip: _____

The next appropriate treatment for this rhythm is:

a. Continue CPR
b. Call the coroner
c. IV and drug therapy
d. Shock at 200 J

Answer: _____

Figure 4-10

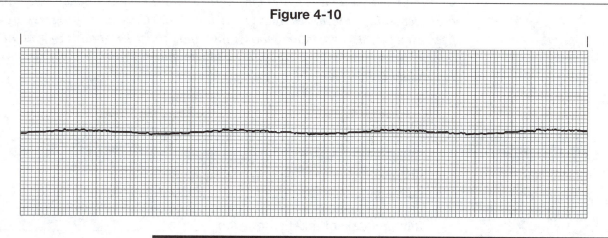

Scenario #11

A 36-year-old male presents with intermittent chest pain that has been present for several days. He came into the ER because his father had a heart attack at the age of 44 and this fact worried the patient. Vital signs are stable and the rhythm in Figure 4-11 is noted after placing him on the cardiac monitor.

Rate: _____

Rhythm: _____

P wave: _____

PRI: _____

QRS: _____

Interpretation of the rhythm strip: _____

Figure 4-11

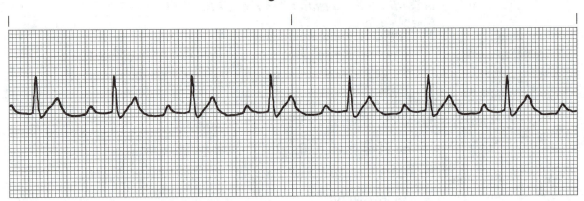

Scenario #12

Emergency Medical Services (EMS) is called to a residence for a patient who reportedly had a seizure. On their arrival at the residence, they find a 58-year-old male unresponsive on the floor. CPR is in progress by a fire/rescue first responder, who stated that the AED had shocked him once. The patient is placed on an EMS monitor, showing the rhythm in Figure 4-12.

Rate: _____

Rhythm: _____

P wave: _____

PRI: _____

QRS: _____

Interpretation of the rhythm strip: _____

Figure 4-12

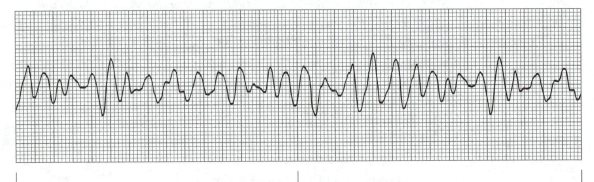

Scenario #13

EMS is called to a residence for a female patient who is having chest pains and shortness of breath. She is conscious but weak; her skin is pale in color and cool and clammy to the touch. Her blood pressure is 70/30, and her heart rate is as noted in the rhythm strip in Figure 4-13. Her respirations are 28 with an oxygen saturation of 88% on room air. The patient is placed on an EMS monitor, showing the rhythm in Figure 4-13.

Rate: _____

Rhythm: _____

P wave: _____

PRI: _____

QRS: _____

Interpretation of the rhythm strip: _____

Figure 4-13

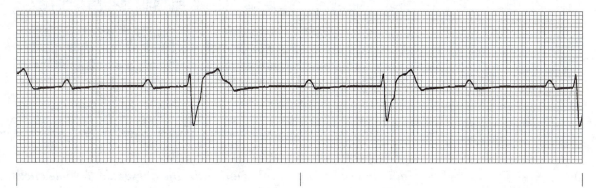

Scenario #14

A patient in the emergency department calls the nurse due to severe chest pain with shortness of breath. The patient's skin is pale, cool, and clammy. Her blood pressure is 80/60, and her heart rate is weak and thready. Her heart rate is as noted in the rhythm in Figure 4-14. Her respirations are 28 with an oxygen saturation of 95% on 2 L of oxygen by nasal cannula. The nurse looks at the monitor and sees the rhythm shown in Figure 4-14.

Rate: _____

Rhythm: _____

P wave: _____

PRI: _____

QRS: _____

Interpretation of the rhythm strip: _____

What is the most appropriate treatment for this patient?

   a. Defibrillation with appropriate biphasic shock
   b. Pharmacologic intervention therapy
   c. Synchronized cardioversion
   d. Vagal maneuvers

Answer: _____

Figure 4-14

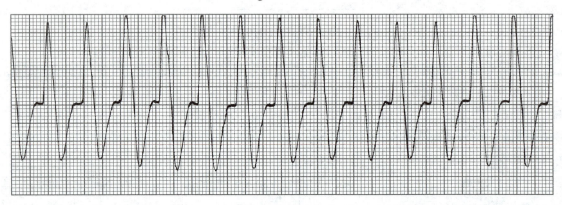

Scenario #15

A patient in the short-stay cardiac unit calls the nurse due to some chest discomfort. The patient's skin is warm, dry, and pink. Blood pressure is 120/80 and the heart rate is noted in Figure 4-15. Respirations are 28 with an

---

Figure 4-15

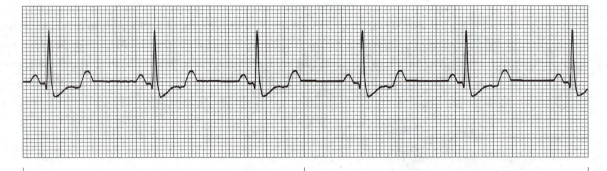

oxygen saturation of 100% on 2 L of oxygen by cannula. The nurse looks at the monitor and sees the rhythm shown in Figure 4-15.

Rate: _____

Rhythm: _____

P wave: _____

PRI: _____

QRS: _____

Interpretation of the rhythm strip: _____

Scenario #16

A patient in the emergency department calls the nurse due to some chest discomfort. The patient's skin is warm, dry to the touch, and pink in color. The patient's blood pressure is 150/77, the heart rate is as noted in Figure 4-16, and the respirations are 28. The oxygen saturation is 100% on 2 L of oxygen by cannula. The nurse looks at the cardiac monitor and sees the rhythm in Figure 4-16.

Rate: _____

Rhythm: _____

P wave: _____

PRI: _____

QRS: _____

Interpretation of the rhythm strip: _____

Figure 4-16

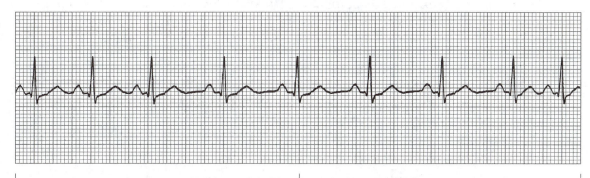

Scenario #17

A patient is picked up at a local physician's office for weakness and short-ness of breath. His skin is warm and dry to the touch and pink in color. His blood pressure is 120/80, and his heart rate is as noted in Figure 4-17. His respirations are 28 with an oxygen saturation at 98% on 2 L of oxygen by nasal cannula.

Rate: _____

Rhythm: _____

P wave: _____

PRI: _____

QRS: _____

Interpretation of the rhythm strip: _____

Figure 4-17

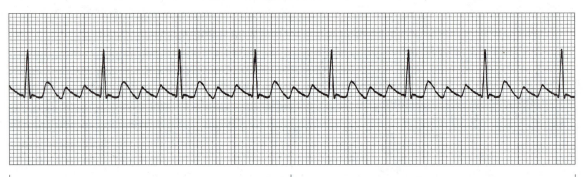

Scenario #18

Mr. Doug Jones calls EMS with complaints of a sudden onset of a fast heart rate and palpations. His skin is pale and cool and moist to the touch. Mr. Jones' blood pressure is 80/66, and his heart rate is as noted in Figure 4-18. His respirations are 28 with an oxygen saturation at 88% on room air.

Rate: _____

Rhythm: _____

P wave: _____

PRI: _____

QRS: _____

Interpretation of the rhythm strip: _____

Figure 4-18

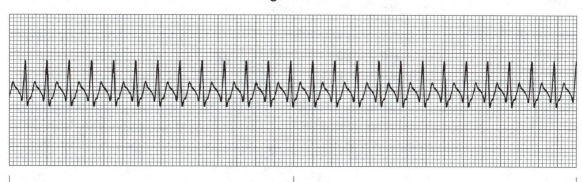

Scenario #19

A nurse in the surgical monitoring room notices a patient's rhythm change. She sees the rhythm in Figure 4-19. Vital signs on the monitoring system are all within normal limits.

Rate: _____

Rhythm: _____

P wave: _____

PRI: _____

QRS: _____

Interpretation of the rhythm strip: _____

Figure 4-19

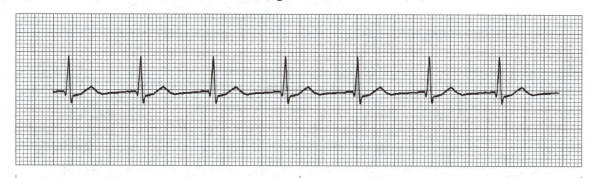

Scenario #20

A patient is brought to the front door of the emergency department, and a family member runs in and says that her father is not breathing. The patient is found unresponsive without heart rate or respirations. The patient is placed in the treatment room and placed on the cardiac monitor, which shows the rhythm in Figure 4-20.

Rate: _____

Rhythm: _____

P wave: _____

PRI: _____

QRS: _____

Interpretation of the rhythm strip: _____

Figure 4-20

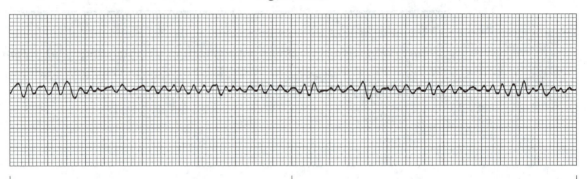

Scenario #21

A patient is brought to the emergency department because he is not feeling well. The patient is complaining of weakness, shortness of breath, and nausea. The patient's skin is cool, pale, and dry to the touch. A cardiac monitor is placed on the patient and shows the rhythm in Figure 4-21.

Figure 4-21

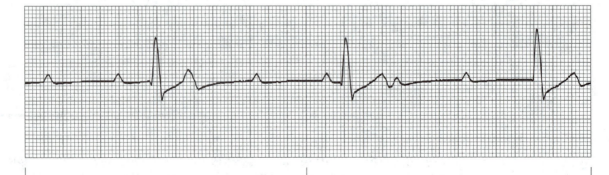

Rate: _____

Rhythm: _____

P wave: _____

PRI: _____

QRS: _____

Interpretation of the rhythm strip: _____

Scenario #22

A woman is brought to the emergency department by EMS because she is not feeling well. The patient is complaining of weakness, shortness of breath, and nausea with vomiting. Her skin is pink, warm, and dry. A cardiac monitor is placed on the patient and shows the rhythm in Figure 4-22.

Rate: _____

Rhythm: _____

P wave: _____

PRI: _____

QRS: _____

Interpretation of the rhythm strip: _____

Figure 4-22

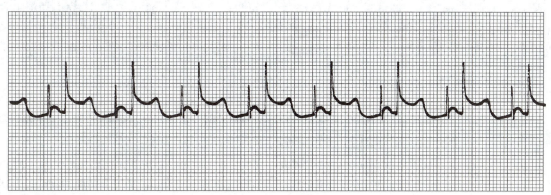

Scenario #23

A patient is brought to the emergency department by ambulance because he was complaining of chest pain that started about 1 hr ago. He is complaining of shortness of breath and nausea with vomiting. The patient's skin is pale, cool, and clammy. A cardiac monitor is placed on the patient and shows the rhythm in Figure 4-23. Then the patient becomes unresponsive and has no pulse.

Rate: _____

Rhythm: _____

P wave: _____

PRI: _____

QRS: _____

Interpretation of the rhythm strip: _____

What is the appropriate treatment for this witnessed rhythm?

a. Pharmacologic intervention
b. Defibrillation with device-specific joules
c. Immediate synchronized cardioversion
d. CPR for 5 min prior to checking heart rate

Answer: _____

Figure 4-23

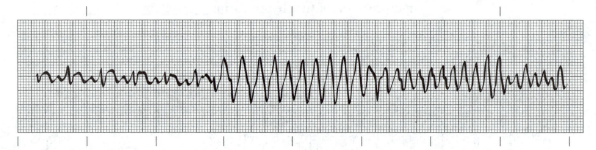

Scenario #24

CPR is in progress with a 67-year-old male patient brought by EMS to the emergency department. The patient has a history of heart disease, based on a verbal report from his granddaughter. This current event included a witnessed rhythm change during transport. The patient is breathing at 10 BPM, and his blood pressure is undetectable. His pulse is absent. The cardiac monitor is now showing the rhythm in Figure 4-24.

Rate: _____

Rhythm: _____

P wave: _____

PRI: _____

QRS: _____

Interpretation of the rhythm strip: _____

Following the 2005 AHA standards, what is the next indicated treatment?

a. Pharmacologic intervention
b. Defibrillation with device-specific joules
c. Immediate synchronized cardioversion
d. Immediate placement of pacemaker

Answer: _____

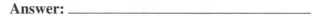

Figure 4-24

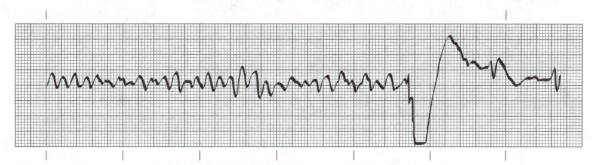

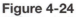

Scenario #25

Mrs. Morrison was brought to the hospital by a fellow member of the local women's study club, where she was in charge of the program for the meeting. She began to complain of "indigestion" immediately after the meeting ended. She took two Rolaids and sat down to rest for 10 min. Although Mrs. Morrison insisted that she felt much better after she belched, her friend insisted that she should go to the hospital. EMS was called, and Mrs. Morrison was transported to the nearest emergency department. She was placed on a cardiac monitor, and the rhythm in Figure 4-25 was noted on the scope. Identify this rhythm, based on the five-step approach.

Rate: _____

Rhythm: _____

P wave: _____

PRI: _____

QRS: _____

Interpretation of the rhythm strip: _____

After a stay of five days, Mrs. Morrison is discharged from the hospital and advised to follow up with a cardiologist within the next week. In this instance, this is appropriate medical care.

    a. True
    b. False

Answer: _____

Figure 4-25

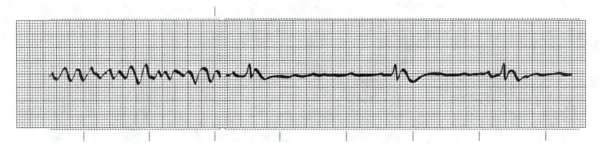

Scenario #26

A 48-year-old female presents to the emergency department with a complaint of pain between the shoulder blades and to her left arm for the last couple of hours. She is also complaining of weakness, shortness of breath, and nausea with vomiting. The patient's skin is pale, warm, and dry. The cardiac monitor is placed on the patient and shows the rhythm in Figure 4-26.

    Rate: _____

    Rhythm: _____

    P wave: _____

Figure 4-26

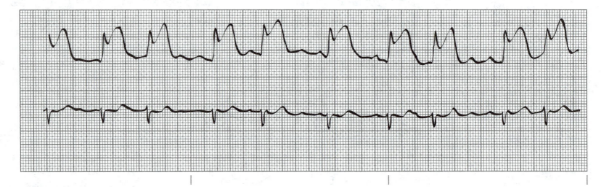

PRI: _____

QRS: _____

Interpretation of the rhythm strip: _____

After giving the patient oxygen at an appropriate amount to keep an oxygen saturation above 95 and ASA 325 mg, what would be the next appropriate treatment for the patient with the rhythm noted in Figure 4-26 per 2005 AHA standards?

    a. Nitroglycerine SL or spray
    b. Heparin
    c. ACE inhibitors
    d. Beta blockers

Answer: _____

Scenario #27

A patient is being monitored in the cardiac observation unit. The patient's skin is pink, warm, and dry. The patient's first and second set of enzymes were within normal limits. The cardiac monitor shows the rhythm in Figure 4-27.

Rate: _____

Rhythm: _____

P wave: _____

PRI: _____

QRS: _____

Interpretation of the rhythm strip: _____

Figure 4-27

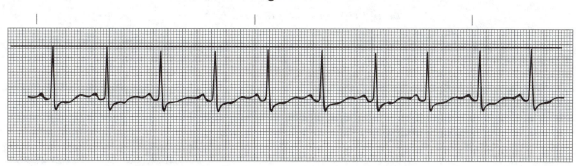

Scenario #28

A 45-year-old male patient is brought to the emergency department by EMS because he was not feeling well. The patient is complaining of weakness, nervousness, and shortness of breath. His skin is pink, warm, and dry. He was seen at his cardiologist's office 4 hrs ago and had a cardiac stress test. The cardiac monitor is placed on the patient and shows the rhythm in Figure 4-28.

Rate: _____

Rhythm: _____

P wave: _____

PRI: _____

QRS: _____

Interpretation of the rhythm strip: _____

Figure 4-28

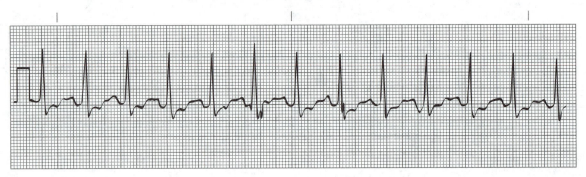

Scenario #29

Mr. Pratt presents to the emergency department, brought by family members because he was not feeling "normal." He is complaining of generalized weakness, mild shortness of breath, and nausea. His skin is cool and clammy to the touch. His blood pressure is 82/60; heart rate is present and is as shown on the rhythm in Figure 4-29.

Rate: _____

Rhythm: _____

P wave: _____

PRI: _____

QRS: _____

Interpretation of the rhythm strip: _____

What is the preferred treatment for this patient with the given symptoms and rhythm?

a. Synchronized cardioversion with appropriate joules
b. Amiodarone
c. Defibrillate with device-specific joules
d. Vasopressor of choice

Answer: _____

Figure 4-29

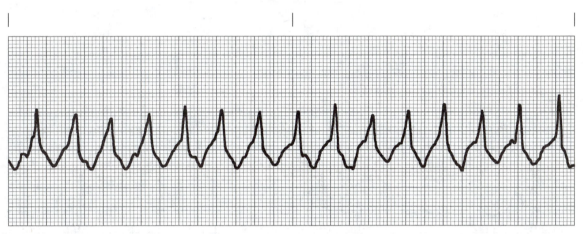

Scenario #30

Mr. Kirby is brought to the emergency department by his coworker because he "would pass out every time he stood up." He is complaining of generalized weakness. His skin is cool, clammy, and pale to touch, with weak distal pulses. The patient is connected to the cardiac monitor and reveals the rhythm shown in Figure 4-30.

Rate: _____

Rhythm: _____

P wave: _____

PRI: _____

QRS: _____

Interpretation of the rhythm strip: _____

The drug of choice in this patient given his symptoms and rhythm is:

a. Transvenous pacer
b. Epinephrine 1 mg 1:10,000 IVP

c. Dopamine infusion at 20 μg/min IVPB

d. Atropine 0.5 mg IVP

Answer: _____

If your first choice does not work, what would be your second choice?

a. Fibrinolytics

b. Vasopressin 40 units IVP

c. Transcutaneous pacer

d. Beta blockers

Answer: _____

Figure 4-30

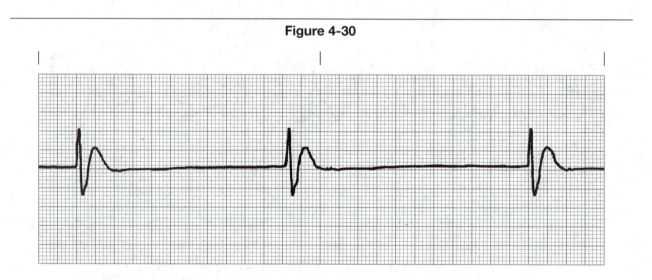

Scenario #31

A patient is brought to the progressive cardiac unit as a direct admit from a physician's office. The patient's skin is pink, warm, and dry. A cardiac monitor is placed on the patient and shows the rhythm in Figure 4-31.

Rate: _____

Rhythm: _____

P wave: _____

PRI: _____

QRS: _____

Interpretation of the rhythm strip: _____

Figure 4-31

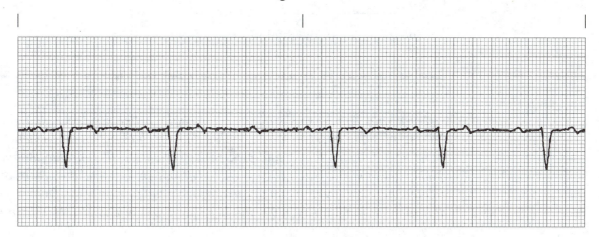

Scenario #32

Mr. Mitchell is a 62-year-old male patient who was picked up by EMS at his residence. He is complaining of sudden onset of chest pain, identifying the pain type as 10 of 10 on the pain scale. He is also complaining of weakness, shortness of breath, and nausea with vomiting. Mr. Mitchell's skin is pale and cool and clammy to the touch. His blood pressure is 122/80, and his heart rate is as noted on the rhythm strip in Figure 4-21, with an oxygen saturation of 95% on room air. A cardiac monitor is placed on the patient and shows the rhythm in Figure 4-32.

Rate: _____

Rhythm: _____

P wave: _____

Figure 4-32

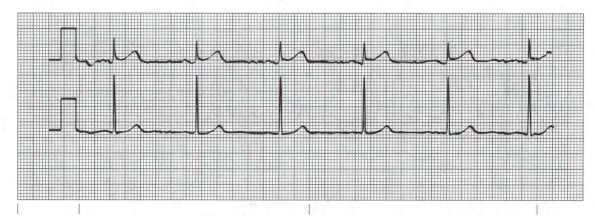

PRI: _____

QRS: _____

Interpretation of the rhythm strip: _____

Scenario #33

A 62-year-old female was sitting in her chair at her residence and complaining of some chest tightness with some shortness of breath when she called 911. EMS responds and places the patient on the cardiac monitor, which shows the rhythm in Figure 4-33. The patient is conscious, alert, and oriented, her skin is warm and dry to the touch and pink in color. Her oxygen saturation on room air is 98%, and her blood pressure is 151/110. Identify the rhythm.

Rate: _____

Rhythm: _____

P wave: _____

PRI: _____

QRS: _____

Interpretation of the rhythm strip: _____

Prehospital initial treatment would be which pharmacological agent?

a. Epi 1 mg/kg IVP
b. Nitroglycerine 0.4 mg SL
c. Amiodarone 150 mg over 10 min IVP
d. Atropine 0.5 mg IVP

Answer: _____

Figure 4-33

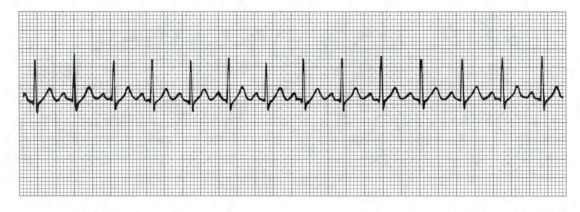

In addition to the initial medication, the patient should also receive:

a. Azomycin
b. Atropine
c. Isuprel
d. Oxygen

Answer: _____

Scenario #34

A patient in the progressive care unit rings the call bell and tells the nurse that she is feeling some "funny feelings" in her chest. She is exhibiting shortness of breath at this time and is pale and cool and clammy to the touch. A cardiac monitor shows the rhythm in Figure 4-34. This rhythm is interpreted as follows.

Rate: _____

Rhythm: _____

P wave: _____

PRI: _____

QRS: _____

Interpretation of the rhythm strip: _____

The problem with this type of ectopic beat is that it can cause:

a. Sustained ventricular fibrillation
b. Postural hypertension
c. Atrial fibrillation
d. Supraventricular tachycardia

Answer: _____

Figure 4-34

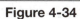
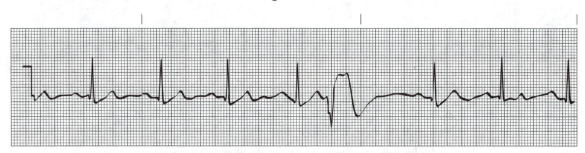

Scenario #35

Mr. Morrison is brought to the emergency department by EMS and is status post arrest. His initial rhythm was apparently ventricular fibrillation or ventricular tachycardia due to fire/rescue utilizing an AED and the patient being defibrillated two times. Advanced Life Support (ALS) arrived and took over the patient's care, continued resuscitation, and transported. The patient has an advanced airway in place and CPR is in progress on arrival. There are no discernible vital signs. The cardiac monitor is placed on the patient and shows the rhythm in Figure 4-35. Based on the case history and the interpretation of the rhythm strip, how would you recognize this rhythm?

Rate: _____

Rhythm: _____

P wave: _____

PRI: _____

QRS: _____

Interpretation of the rhythm strip: _____

You recognize that this patient is experiencing:

a. Post shock syndrome
b. Asystole
c. PEA

Answer: _____

Figure 4-35

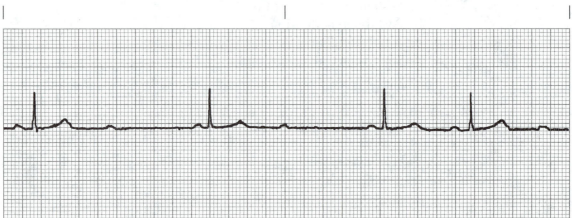

Scenario #36

Mr. Brown was midway through his brisk morning walk when he began to experience mild chest discomfort. He denies that the pain radiates and states that it is located "behind his breastbone."

Mr. Brown states that he takes vitamins each day and no other meds. He reports no allergies. He also states that he felt much better when he went home and rested for a while. His vital signs are as follows: blood pressure, 140/88; heart rate, 76; respiration, 22 breaths per minute. His skin is warm and dry to the touch. Identify his rhythm as it appears in the strip in Figure 4-36.

Rate: _____

Rhythm: _____

P wave: _____

PRI: _____

QRS: _____

Interpretation of the rhythm strip: _____

Figure 4-36

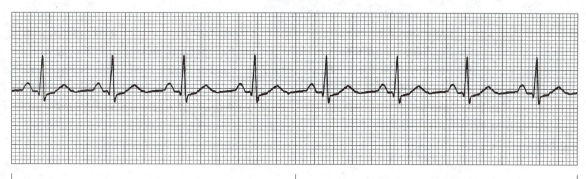

Scenario #37

Your patient, Mrs. Johnson, is a 74-year-old female who reports a long history of "heart problems." However, she also states that she has not undergone any heart surgery. She is complaining of shortness of breath that becomes much worse when she goes from her bedroom to her kitchen. Upon initial exam, she is noted to have bilateral rales in both lower lobes as well as +1 pitting edema. Her medications are: Digitalis, once daily, and Diovan, 60 mg daily. She is placed on a monitor, and her ECG strip shows the rhythm in Figure 4-37.

Rate: _____

Rhythm: _____

P wave: _____

PRI: _____

QRS: _____

Interpretation of the rhythm strip: _____

Figure 4-37

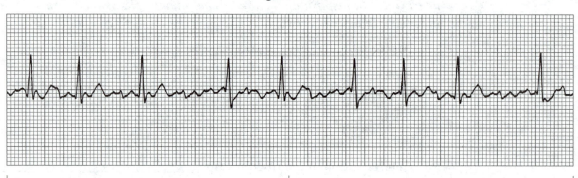

Scenario #38

Mr. Duke is an 87-year-old male patient who lives alone. He activates his Lifeline, and when EMS arrives, he is slumped over in the bathroom, sitting on the toilet. He responds to verbal stimuli, his skin is pale, cool, and clammy, and he denies any pain. Mr. Duke is moved to the gurney, and he has an IV established and is connected to a cardiac monitor. See Figure 4-38.

Rate: _____

Rhythm: _____

P wave: _____

PRI: _____

QRS: _____

Interpretation of the rhythm strip: _____

Figure 4-38

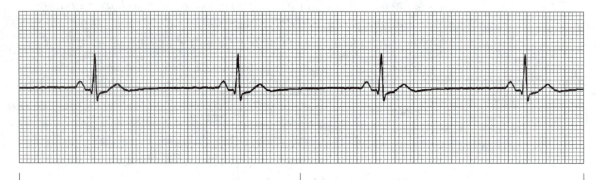

Your initial pharmacological treatment for Mr. Duke should be:

a. Lidocaine, 200 mg IVP
b. Nitroglycerine, 0.12 mg SL
c. Oxygen at 15 L via NRM
d. Atropine, 0.025 IV

Answer: _____

Scenario #39

EMS is called to the scene of a middle-aged man who reportedly is having a seizure. The first responder finds him unresponsive, pulseless, and apneic. CPR is initiated prior to the arrival of ALS. When ALS arrives on the scene, they take control of the scene and initiate an advanced airway and place the patient on the cardiac monitor. The rhythm in Figure 4-39 is shown on the monitor.

Rate: _____

Rhythm: _____

P wave: _____

PRI: _____

QRS: _____

Interpretation of the rhythm strip: _____

After the initial shock is delivered and 2 min of CPR is provided, the rhythm is unchanged. The appropriate ALS pharmachal therapy is:

a. Epinephrine, 4.0 mg IVP
b. Vasopressin, 40 units IVP
c. Amiodarone, 300 mg IVP
d. Atropine, 0.5 mg IVP

Answer: _____

Figure 4-39

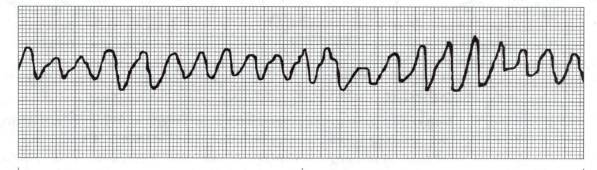

Scenario #40

Billy is a 40-year-old male who arrived at the emergency department complaining of dizziness and shortness of breath. The ER nurse noticed that the patient was diaphoretic and pale. She places him in a wheelchair and takes him to a treatment room. Billy's vital signs are taken as he is being placed on the monitor. His blood pressure is 70/40, his heart rate is rapid and weak, and he is respiring at 32 breaths per minute. The cardiac monitor shows the rhythm in Figure 4-40.

Rate: _____

Rhythm: _____

P wave: _____

PRI: _____

QRS: _____

Interpretation of the rhythm strip: _____

Since Billy is hemodynamically unstable, the appropriate therapy is:

a. Defibrillation at 100 J
b. Cardioversion at 100 J
c. Administer 4 mg MS IM
d. Carotid sinus massage

Answer: _____

Figure 4-40

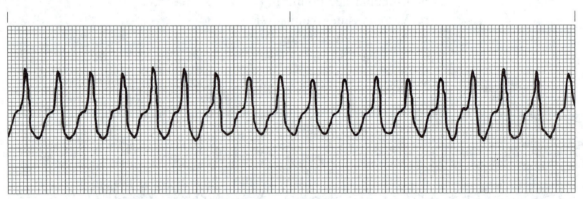

Scenario #41

Ginger is a 52-year-old female with a past medical history of IDDM who presents to her doctor's office complaining of shortness of breath and feeling tired for one day. She denies any chest pain, but is having pain to the left arm and neck. On assessment, the physician finds that she has bilateral rales in the lower lobes and is slightly hypotensive with a blood pressure of 88/56. He calls EMS and, on their arrival, places her on a cardiac monitor, which shows the rhythm in Figure 4-41.

Rate: _____

Rhythm: _____

P wave: _____

PRI: _____

QRS: _____

Interpretation of the rhythm strip: _____

Due to the findings on this ECG, the appropriate ALS therapy for this rhythm is:

a. Morphine, 2 mg IVP
b. Nitroglycerine, 0.04 mg SL
c. 12-lead EKG
d. External pacer

Answer: _____

Figure 4-41

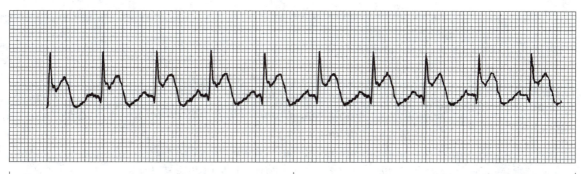

Scenario #42

Mr. Williams, a 65-year-old male, presents to the emergency department with the complaint of not feeling well and is tired all the time. He does have a past history of ASHD and is on Digitalis, 0.025 mg daily. Vital signs are assessed, showing an initial BP of 120/66, heart rate as listed on the rhythm shown in Figure 4-42, and respirations at 22 times a minute with an oxygen saturation of 91% on room air. He is placed on the cardiac monitor, which shows the rhythm in Figure 4-42.

Rate: _____

Rhythm: _____

P wave: _____

PRI: _____

QRS: _____

Interpretation of the rhythm strip: _____

Figure 4-42

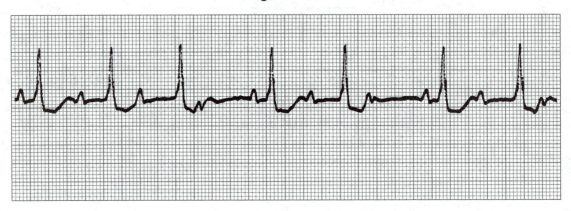

Scenario #43

Ms. Jones calls 911 for her father, who is complaining of shortness of breath and near syncope every time he gets up from the couch. On arrival of EMS, they assess Mr. Jones and find that he is cool, clammy, and pale and that he responds to verbal stimuli only. He is placed on nonrebreather mask at 15 liters per minute and a cardiac monitor. Vital signs are also taken, showing a blood pressure of 50/pal; respirations are 28 and slightly labored. The cardiac monitor shows the rhythm in Figure 4-43.

Figure 4-43

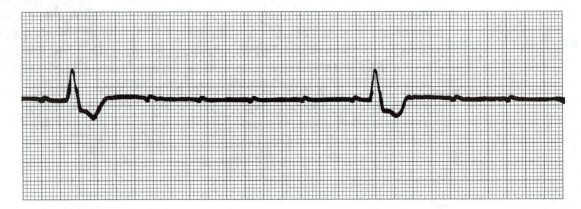

Rate: _____

Rhythm: _____

P wave: _____

PRI: _____

QRS: _____

Interpretation of the rhythm strip: _____

With this rhythm, the appropriate ALS therapy is:

  a. Immediate CPR and intubation
  b. Immediate defibrillation
  c. Immediate cardioversion
  d. Immediate external cardiac pacing

Answer: _____

Scenario #44

Mr. Jackson was out working in his yard when he started having some chest pain radiating to his left arm. He stopped working, went into the house, and sat on the couch. His wife gave him a nitroglycerine SL. She also called 911 for EMS. EMS arrived to find Mr. Jackson feeling somewhat better with the pain almost gone. Mr. Jackson states, however, that he is still feeling some "funny feelings" in his chest like his heart is "skipping a beat." EMS connects the patient to the cardiac monitor, showing the rhythm in Figure 4-44.

Rate: _____

Rhythm: _____

P wave: _____

PRI: _____

QRS: _____

Interpretation of the rhythm strip: _____

Figure 4-44

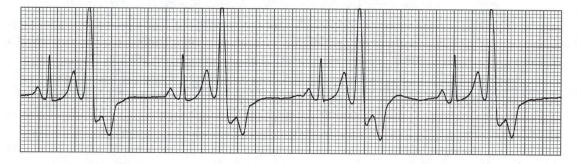

Scenario #45

Mrs. Taylor is 42-year-old female who presented to the walk-in clinic with a sudden onset of chest pain after having an argument with her husband. She has a history of mitral valve prolapse. Her blood pressure is 116/80, her heart rate is as stated in Figure 4-45, and respirations are 22 and nonlabored. She is placed on a cardiac monitor, showing the rhythm in Figure 4-45.

Rate: _____

Rhythm: _____

P wave: _____

PRI: _____

QRS: _____

Interpretation of the rhythm strip: _____

Figure 4-45

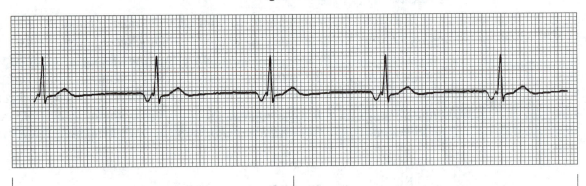

Scenario #46

Mrs. White is an 80-year-old female who is quite active, considering her age. Her favorite pastime is working in her garden, in particular, planting and growing petunias. She has a history of "heart trouble" but has done quite well and continues to live alone. One bright summer day, she is busily weeding her garden when she begins to "feel funny." She calls her daughter, who immediately takes her to the emergency department. Her vital signs are found to be: blood pressure,140/90; heart rate as demonstrated on the rhythm strip in Figure 4-46; and respiratory rate, 20 breaths per minute. What is her rhythm?

Rate: _____

Rhythm: _____

P wave: _____

PRI: _____

QRS: _____

Interpretation of the rhythm strip: _____

Figure 4-46

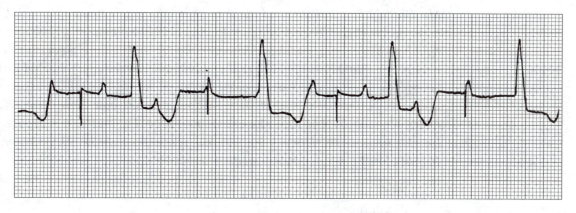

Scenario #47

Ms. Wright, a 77-year-old female, came in a taxi to the emergency department because she was "feeling very weak" and just thought she needed to be checked by the doctor. Ms. Wright was placed in an assessment room and her vital signs were found to be: blood pressure, 100/60; heart rate as shown on the rhythm strip in Figure 4-47; and respirations, 18 breaths per minute. Identify her rhythm.

Rate: _____

Rhythm: _____

P wave: _____

Figure 4-47

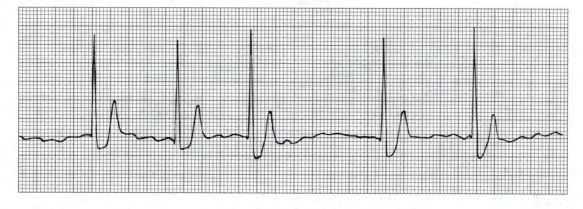

PRI: _____

QRS: _____

Interpretation of the rhythm strip: _____

Scenario #48

Mr. Blakely is a 58-year-old male patient who was attending a neighbor-hood party when a friend told him to play a joke on another friend and pre-tend he was snorting cocaine. However, the "friend" put real cocaine on the mirror. Mr. Blakely sniffed the real cocaine and immediately started experiencing chest pain. EMS was called to the scene and began to assess and treat this patient. His vital signs were found to be: blood pressure, 92/58; heart rate as seen in the rhythm in Figure 4-48, and respiration of 28 breaths per minute. His oxygen saturation is reported as 88% on room air. Identify Mr. Blakely's rhythm strip.

Rate: _____

Rhythm: _____

P wave: _____

PRI: _____

QRS: _____

Interpretation of the rhythm strip: _____

After initial treatment with oxygen and IV therapy, the pharmacological intervention for this rhythm should be:

a. Procainamide, 10 mg IVP
b. Amiodarone, 300 mg IVB
c. Adenosine, 6 mg IVP
d. Atropine, 0.4 mg IVB

Answer: _____

Figure 4-48

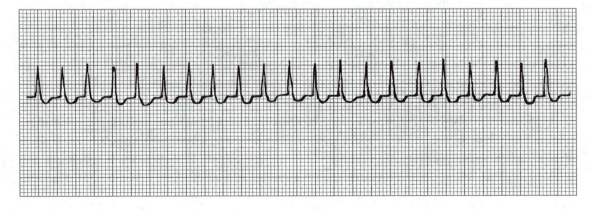

Scenario #49

Mr. Moore was brought to the emergency department by his daughter and presented to the ambulance doors unresponsive in the passenger seat. The nurses assessed that he was unresponsive, without a pulse, and apneic, and they called for the paramedics to assist in transporting the patient into the emergency department. After placing Mr. Moore on the treatment bed, CPR was initiated while placing the patient on the monitor. The monitor illustrated the rhythm in Figure 4-49. Identify the rhythm.

Rate: _____

Rhythm: _____

P wave: _____

PRI: _____

QRS: _____

Interpretation of the rhythm strip: _____

Figure 4-49

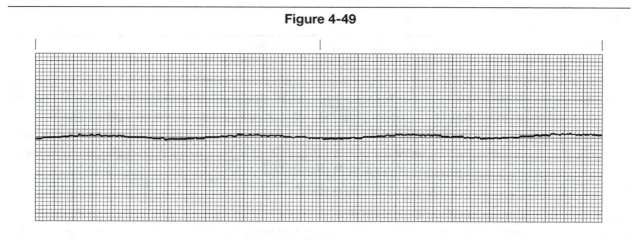

Scenario #50

Mr. Boone is a 69-year-old male patient who is complaining of persistent fatigue for more than 2 days. He states that he has no significant past medical history and he takes no medications other than vitamins and occasional antacids. His vital signs are within normal limits. His oxygen saturation is 97% on room air. The monitor illustrated the rhythm in Figure 4-50. Identify his rhythm.

Rate: _____

Rhythm: _____

P wave: _____

PRI: _____

QRS: _____

Interpretation of the rhythm strip: _____

Figure 4-50

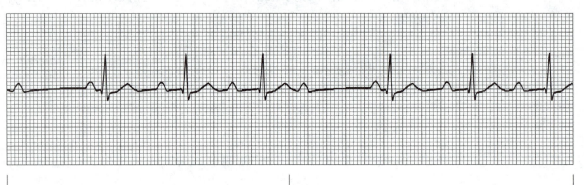

Scenario #51

A 12-year-old female is brought to the emergency room with dizziness that started after taking some "pills" at a friends' house. The medication is determined to be a grandparent's Digitalis. Her blood pressure is 80/54, pulse is as shown in Figure 4-51, and respirations are 24 with an oxygen saturation on room air of 95%. You place the patient on the cardiac monitor, and it shows the rhythm in Figure 4-51.

Figure 4-51

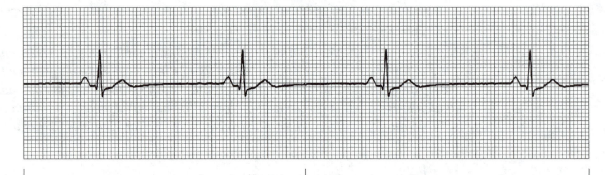

Rate: _____

Rhythm: _____

P wave: _____

PRI: _____

QRS: _____

Interpretation of the rhythm strip: _____

Scenario #52

A 36-year-old female comes to her doctor's office with weakness for a few days. She stated that she has been taking a blood pressure pill that "a friend" had given to her for the past several days. The nurse checks her blood pressure; it is 70/40, her pulse is as depicted in Figure 4-52, and her oxygen saturation on room air is 95%. An ambulance is called, and on its arrival at the doctor's office, the patient is placed on the cardiac monitor. It shows the rhythm in Figure 4-52.

Rate: _____

Rhythm: _____

P wave: _____

PRI: _____

QRS: _____

Interpretation of the rhythm strip: _____

Figure 4-52

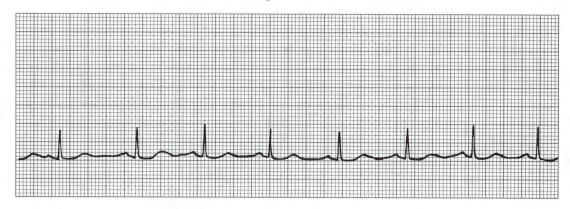

Scenario #53

A 35-year-old male presents to the emergency department with chest pain that started after taking some "cocaine" for the first time. His blood pressure is 170/99; his pulse is as shown in Figure 4-53. His respirations are 24, with oxygen saturation on room air of 95%. You place the patient on the cardiac monitor, and it shows the rhythm in Figure 4-53.

Rate: _____

Rhythm: _____

P wave: _____

PRI: _____

QRS: _____

Interpretation of the rhythm strip: _____

Figure 4-53

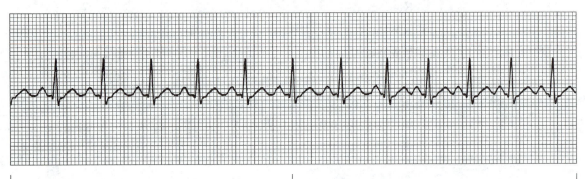

Scenario #54

A 59-year-old female calls 911 requesting an ambulance and complaining of "feeling like her heart stops." The ambulance staff arrives, and the assessments reveals a blood pressure of 140/90, a pulse as shown in Figure 4-54, and respirations of 22 with an oxygen saturation on room air of 97%. She is placed on the cardiac monitor, and it shows the rhythm in Figure 4-54.

Rate: _____

Rhythm: _____

P wave: _____

PRI: _____

QRS: _____

Interpretation of the rhythm strip: _____

Figure 4-54

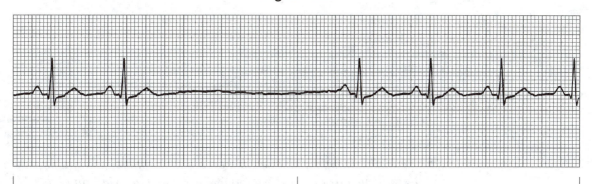

Scenario #55

A 76-year-old male presents to the emergency department with a complaint of "an irregular heart beat" since this morning. His blood pressure is 130/88, his pulse is as shown in Figure 4-55, and his respirations are 22 with an oxygen saturation on room air of 97%. You place the patient on the cardiac monitor, and it shows the rhythm in Figure 4-55.

Rate: _____

Rhythm: _____

P wave: _____

Figure 4-55

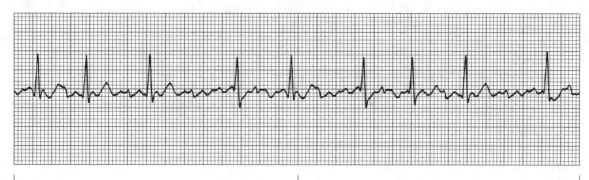

PRI: _____

QRS: _____

Interpretation of the rhythm strip: _____

What medication would most likely be utilized to convert the rhythm?

a. Atropine
b. Lidocaine
c. Cardiozem
d. Adenosine

Answer: _____

Scenario #56

A 53-year-old female presents at her doctor's office and states that she "thinks that she has been taking too much of her Lanoxin" and has not been feeling well. Her blood pressure is 100/76. Her pulse is as shown in Figure 4-56, and her respirations are 24 with an oxygen saturation on room air of 96%. An ambulance is called to the office. They place the patient on the cardiac monitor, and it shows the rhythm in Figure 4-56.

Rate: _____

Rhythm: _____

P wave: _____

PRI: _____

QRS: _____

Interpretation of the rhythm strip: _____

Figure 4-56

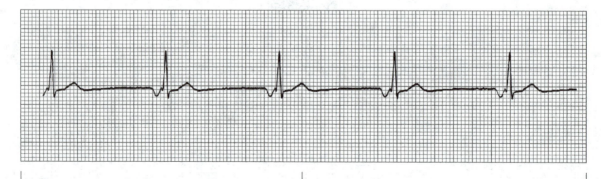

Scenario #57

A 45-year-old male presents to the emergency department and states, "I think my heart is having skipped beats," which makes him feel funny. His blood pressure is 138/76, his pulse is as in Figure 4-57, and his respirations are 24 with an oxygen saturation on room air of 96%. You place the patient on the cardiac monitor, and it shows the rhythm in Figure 4-57.

Rate: _____

Rhythm: _____

P wave: _____

PRI: _____

QRS: _____

Interpretation of the rhythm strip: _____

Figure 4-57

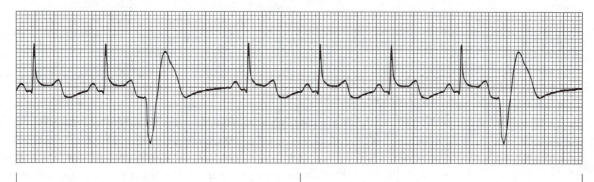

Scenario #58

A 45-year-old male pushes the call button from his bed in the cardiac short-stay unit and stated that "the feeling of the skipped beats in my chest is getting worse." The patient's blood pressure is 122/70. His pulse is as shown In Figure 4-58, and his respirations are 24 with an oxygen saturation on room air of 96%. You look at the cardiac monitor and see the rhythm in Figure 4-58.

Rate: _____

Rhythm: _____

P wave: _____

PRI: _____

QRS: _____

Interpretation of the rhythm strip: _____

Would you give this patient any medication to stop the ectopic beats?

   a. Yes
   b. No

Answer: _____

Figure 4-58

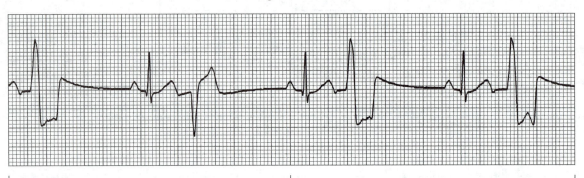

Scenario #59

A 55-year-old male becomes unresponsive sitting at the triage desk in the emergency department and slumps over. The patient is placed on a stretcher and rolled into a treatment room. He is not breathing and does not have a pulse. CPR is started while you place the patient on the cardiac monitor. It shows the rhythm in Figure 4-59.

Figure 4-59

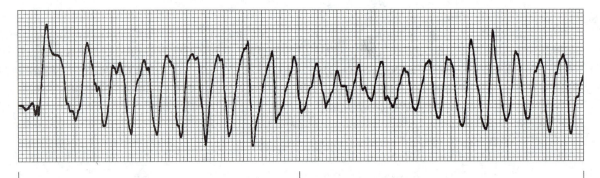

Rate: _____

Rhythm: _____

P wave: _____

PRI: _____

QRS: _____

Interpretation of the rhythm strip: _____

Scenario #60

Mr. Kelly is visiting his wife in the hospital and is found unresponsive, sitting in a chair. Mr. Kelly is placed on a stretcher. He is not breathing and does not have a pulse. He is placed on the cardiac monitor, and it showed a ventricular fibrillation rhythm. The patient is defibrillated with the appropriate joules, and the rhythm in Figure 4-60 is noted on the cardiac monitor after 2 min of CPR.

Rate: _____

Rhythm: _____

P wave: _____

PRI: _____

QRS: _____

Interpretation of the rhythm strip: _____

Figure 4-60

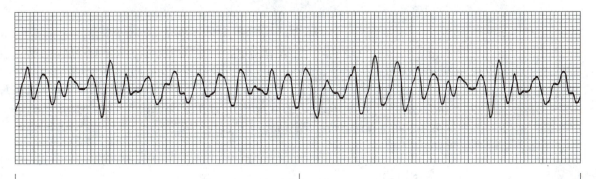

Scenario #61

Mr. Brick, a 36-year-old male, presents to his doctor's office with intermittent chest pain for the past 5 days. He came in because his father had a heart attack at the age of 38 and, based on this history, he was worried about the pain. His vital signs are stable and, when the ECG is recorded, his physician notes the rhythm in Figure 4-61.

Rate: _____

Rhythm: _____

P wave: _____

PRI: _____

QRS: _____

Interpretation of the rhythm strip: _____

Figure 4-61

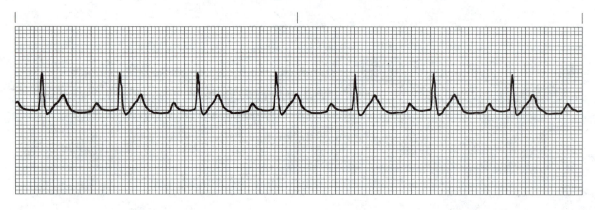

Scenario #62

Emergency medical services is called to a residence for a patient who has had a seizure. On their arrival at the residence, they find Mr. Howard, a 58-year-old male, lying unresponsive on the floor in a supine position. CPR is in progress by a fire/rescue first responder, who stated that the AED had shocked the patient once. The patient is placed on an EMS cardiac monitor; the monitor reveals the rhythm in Figure 4-62.

Rate: _____

Rhythm: _____

P wave: _____

PRI: _____

QRS: _____

Interpretation of the rhythm strip: _____

Figure 4-62

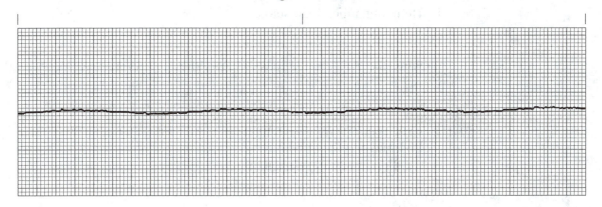

Scenario #63

EMS is called to Mr. Mitchum's residence when his wife reports that he is sick. On their arrival at the residence, they find a 55-year-old male lying on the couch complaining of chest pain. His skin is cool and clammy, and he is pale in color. His initial blood pressure is 88/40; his pulse rate is rapid and regular. Mr. Mitchum is placed on the EMS cardiac monitor, and the medics note the rhythm in Figure 4-63.

Rate: _____

Rhythm: _____

P wave: _____

Figure 4-63

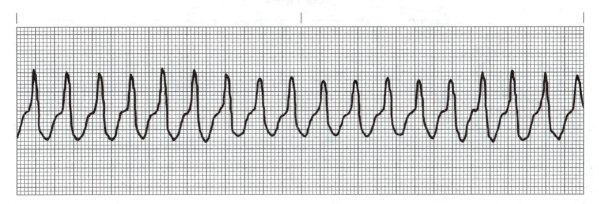

PRI: _____

QRS: _____

Interpretation of the rhythm strip: _____

In this scenario with the listed rhythm, the patient is: _____.

    a. Hemodynamically stable
    b. Hemodynamically unstable

Answer: _____

Following the AHA guidelines, what is the appropriate treatment for this rhythm?

    a. Immediate defibrillation
    b. Synchronized cardioversion
    c. Pharmacologic intervention
    d. Cardiopulmonary resuscitation.

Answer: _____

Scenario #64

Mrs. Brown in a 48-year-old female who is admitted to the monitored floor from a doctor's office. She is complaining of weakness, dizziness, and a slow pulse. The nurse places the patient in a bed, and on the cardiac monitor, which shows the rhythm in Figure 4-64.

Rate: _____

Rhythm: _____

P wave: _____

PRI: _____

QRS: _____

Interpretation of the rhythm strip: _____

Figure 4-64

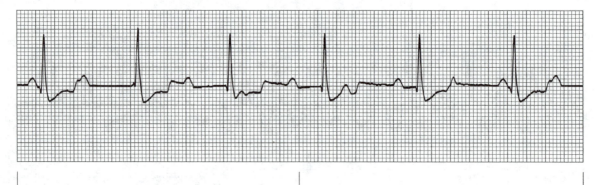

Scenario #65

EMS is called to a residence for a patient complaining of problems with balance and dizziness. They find Mr. Boone, who is a 68-year-old male sitting in the couch attended by a fire/rescue first responder. Mr. Boone is placed on an EMS monitor, and the rhythm in Figure 4-65 is observed.

Rate: _____

Rhythm: _____

P wave: _____

PRI: _____

QRS: _____

Interpretation of the rhythm strip: _____

Figure 4-65

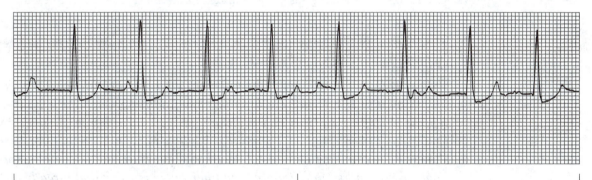

Scenario #66

A large urban EMS service is summoned to respond to a small outlying rural hospital to transfer a patient to the cardiac center for the regional area. At the transferring emergency department, they find Mr. Bartlett, a 68-year-old male, sitting on a cot in a treatment room. Mr. Bartlett is conversable and alert. He reports to you that he was watching a football game at home and suddenly began to feel a "strange" sensation in his chest. His vital signs are within normal limits, and his monitor shows the rhythm in Figure 4-66.

Rate: _____

Rhythm: _____

P wave: _____

PRI: _____

QRS: _____

Interpretation of the rhythm strip: _____

Figure 4-66

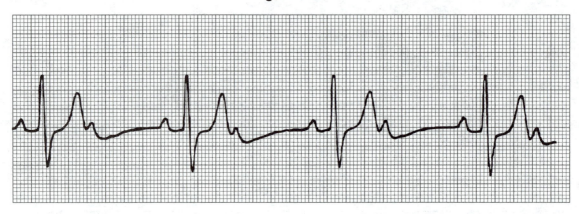

Scenario #67

EMS is called to a residence for a patient who was experiencing difficulty breathing and substernal chest pain. They find a 65-year-old female who reports her name as Gert and is sitting on the couch, being attended by a fire/rescue first responder. The patient is placed on an EMS monitor, which shows the rhythm in Figure 4-67. Her blood pressure is 78/40, her respirations are 28 and slightly labored, and her pulse is weak and thready at the rate shown in the figure. What is the rhythm?

Rate: _____

Rhythm: _____

Figure 4-67

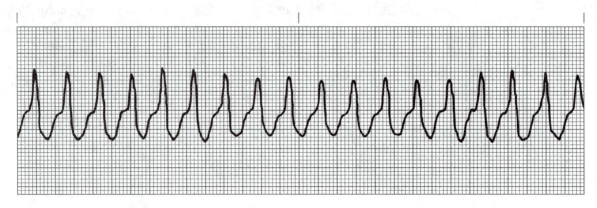

P wave: _____

PRI: _____

QRS: _____

Interpretation of the rhythm strip: _____

This patient falls into the category of hemodynamically unstable. The preferred AHA guidelines suggest that the treatment should be:

a. Drug therapy
b. Immediate defibrillation
c. Synchronized cardioversion
d. Immediate transport

Answer: _____

Scenario #68

Mr. Stephens, a 41-year-old male, presents to the emergency department with a complaint of a "funny feeling" in his chest for the past several days. It comes and goes but has been getting worse this morning. His blood pressure is 180/88, his respirations are 22, and his heart rate is as shown in Figure 4-68. Mr. Stephens is placed on a cardiac monitor, and it shows the rhythm in Figure 4-68.

Rate: _____

Rhythm: _____

P wave: _____

PRI: _____

QRS: _____

Interpretation of the rhythm strip: _____

Figure 4-68

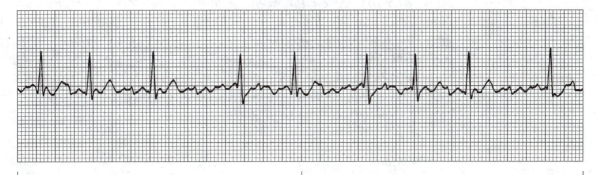

Scenario #69

EMS is called to the airport for a patient experiencing problems with dizziness. They find a 58-year-old male flight attendant sitting in baggage claim and being attended by a fire/rescue first responder. Mr. Bunn, the patient, has just completed a transatlantic flight and states he is exhausted. He is placed on an EMS cardiac monitor, which shows the rhythm in Figure 4-69.

Rate: _____

Rhythm: _____

P wave: _____

PRI: _____

QRS: _____

Interpretation of the rhythm strip: _____

Figure 4-69

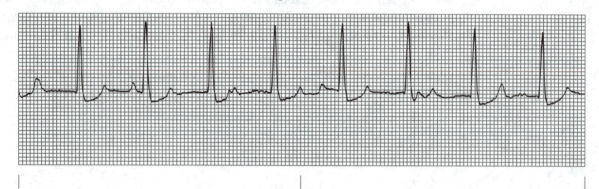

Scenario #70

Mr. Jones is attending the company picnic at the local park when he suddenly clutches his chest and falls to the ground. His wife calls 911 immediately. ALS arrives on the scene within 3 min. Mrs. Jones informs the paramedics that Mr. Jones is 3 months post-op from quadruple bypass surgery. She also informs the medics that Mr. Jones is a Certified Registered Nurse Anesthetist. Mr. Jones is assessed, and his vital signs are: blood pressure, 136/86; heart rate, 72; and respirations, 24. His oxygen saturation is 92% without supplemental oxygen. He is alert and cooperative. Identify his rhythm, as illustrated in Figure 4-70.

Rate: _____

Rhythm: _____

P wave: _____

PRI: _____

QRS: _____

Interpretation of the rhythm strip: _____

Figure 4-70

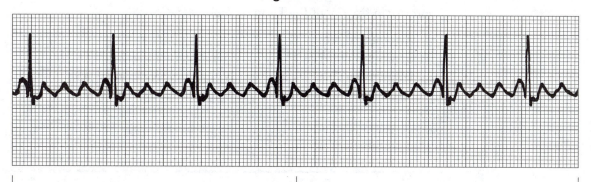

Scenario #71

Thomas Walker is a 38-year-old male patient who has decided to take up running as his form of exercise. He elects to make his first run a 2-mi trek around the local football field. After about ½ mi, Thomas begins to pant, and he elects to run only 1 mi today. Just as he approaches the ¾-mi marker, he begins to feel extreme nausea and faintness. Thomas stops, walks to a shaded tree, and sits down. He is very pale in appearance and is cool and clammy to the touch. A passerby sees Thomas sitting by the tree and immediately calls 911. When the paramedics arrive on the scene and place Thomas on a cardiac monitor, they see the rhythm in Figure 4-71. Identify the rhythm.

Figure 4-71

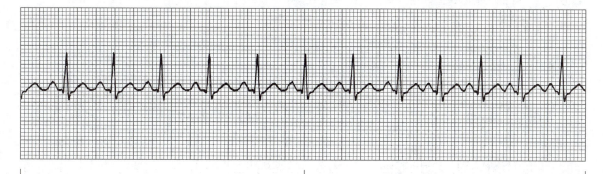

Rate: _____

Rhythm: _____

P wave: _____

PRI: _____

QRS: _____

Interpretation of the rhythm strip: _____

Appropriate treatment for Thomas includes:

   a. Atropine, 0.4 mg IM
   b. Oxygen therapy at 15 LPM; nonrebreather mask
   c. Transport to health care facility for immediate stress test
   d. Consider immediate endotracheal intubation

Answer: _____

Scenario #72

Mr. Crawford presents to his doctor's office and states that he has not been feeling well since he got his last prescription of Digitalis filled and began to take it. He hands the prescription bottle to the doctor, who immediately checks the label and begins to frown as he determines that the pharmacy has dispensed an incorrect dosage of the prescribed medication. The doctor places Mr. Crawford on the cardiac monitor and notes the rhythm in Figure 4-72.

Rate: _____

Rhythm: _____

P wave: _____

Figure 4-72

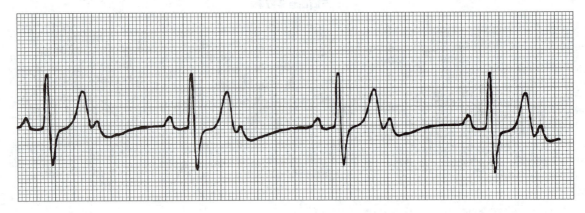

PRI: _____

QRS: _____

Interpretation of the rhythm strip: _____

Mr. Crawford's problem was most likely caused by:

a. Noncompliance
b. Pharmacy error
c. Physician error
d. Lack of patient education

Answer: _____

Scenario #73

EMS is called to a residence for a possible overdose. Mr. Samford, a 28-year-old male, was found unresponsive by his roommate. The roommate found empty pill bottles that were labeled as Valium and Xanax. There is also an empty vodka bottle in the room. Mr. Samford is unresponsive and breathing shallowly. First responders arrive on the scene and immediately phone for paramedic assistance. They begin to assist respirations with a bag-valve-mask. The ALS unit arrives and places the cardiac monitor on the patient. The rhythm is shown in Figure 4-73. Identify the rhythm.

Rate: _____

Rhythm: _____

P wave: _____

PRI: _____

QRS: _____

Interpretation of the rhythm strip: _____

Figure 4-73

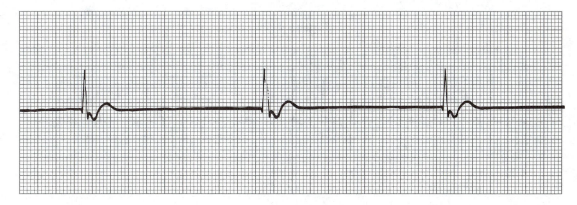

The appropriate pharmacologic intervention would be:

a. Procainamide
b. Epinephrine
c. Atropine
d. Adenosine

Answer: _____

Scenario #74

Mrs. Jenkins is a 79-year-old female patient who called her son because she was not feeling well. After his arrival, he called 911 because she was experiencing difficulty breathing. Paramedics arrive on the scene to find her conscious and oriented to person, place, and time. Her skin is cool and clammy to the touch and appears a bit pale in color. Her distal pulses are rapid and weak to palpation. Identify Mrs. Jenkins' heart rhythm, as noted in Figure 4-74, when she was placed on the cardiac monitor.

Rate: _____

Rhythm: _____

P wave: _____

PRI: _____

QRS: _____

Interpretation of the rhythm strip: _____

The appropriate initial pharmacologic intervention for this patient is:

a. Adenosine, 6 mg IV
b. Adenosine, 12 mg IV
c. Adenosine, 6 mg IM
d. Adenosine, 0.12 mg IV

Answer: _____

Figure 4-74

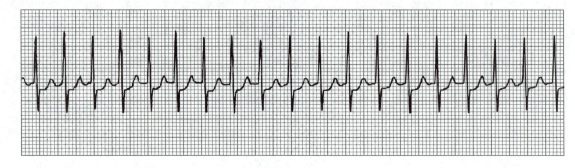

Scenario #75

Mr. Steele is a 48-year-old business executive who reports a history of hypertension. He is at his office when he starts having chest pains after assessing the day's stock market report. His pain is described as "substernal, with radiation to his neck and left jaw." His secretary calls 911, and the paramedics quickly arrive on the scene. He reports his medications as Lopressor, and he also takes baby aspirin (81 mg) and Viagra, as indicated. His vital signs are: blood pressure, 100/88; heart rate as noted on the rhythm in Figure 4-75; respiration, 26 breaths per minute. His skin is ashen in color and is cool and clammy to the touch. Identify his rhythm.

Rate: _____

Rhythm: _____

P wave: _____

PRI: _____

QRS: _____

Interpretation of the rhythm strip: _____

Which of the following medications would be contraindicated for Mr. Steele's chest pain?

   a. Morphine sulfate
   b. Nitroglycerine
   c. Tordal
   d. Demerol

Answer: _____

Figure 4-75

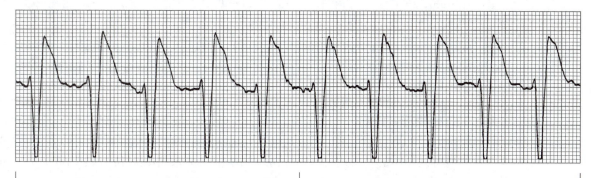

Scenario #76

Mr. Payne is a 56-year-old male who was working in his yard this morning and started to have chest pain. He has a past medical history of hypertension and is on HCTZ daily. He stops working in the yard, goes into the house, and tells his wife. She calls 911 and the paramedics quickly arrive on the scene. His vital signs are: blood pressure, 130/88; heart rate as noted on the rhythm in Figure 4-76; respiration, 26 breaths per minute. His skin is ashen in color and is cool and clammy to the touch. Identify his rhythm.

Rate: _____

Rhythm: _____

P wave: _____

PRI: _____

QRS: _____

Interpretation of the rhythm strip: _____

Which of the following medications would be indicated for Mr. Payne's chest pain?

a. Morphine sulfate
b. Nitroglycerine
c. Hydrocodone
d. Demerol

Answer: _____

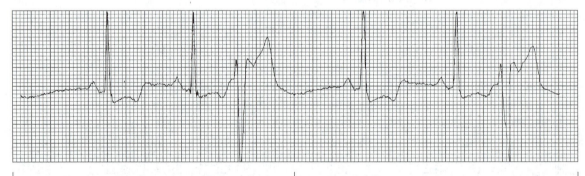

Figure 4-76

Scenario #77

Mrs. Marable, a 65-year-old female, is raking leaves in her front yard one bright spring day. She is reminiscing about the lovely birthday party that her daughter had given her yesterday, when suddenly she begins to experience "tightness" in her chest, and she feels faint. She goes to her front porch and uses her cell phone to call 911. The paramedics arrive on scene and begin their assessment of Mrs. Marable. Her vital signs are: blood pressure, 144/86; heart rate as shown in Figure 4-77. She is respiring at a rate of 26 breaths per minute and her oxygen saturation is 97% on 6 L of oxygen. Identify the ECG rhythm strip.

Rate: _____

Rhythm: _____

P wave: _____

PRI: _____

QRS: _____

Interpretation of the rhythm strip: _____

Which of the following interventions would be appropriate for Mrs. Marable's condition?

   a. Oxygen
   b. Demerol IM
   c. Morphine
   d. Valium

Answer: _____

Figure 4-77

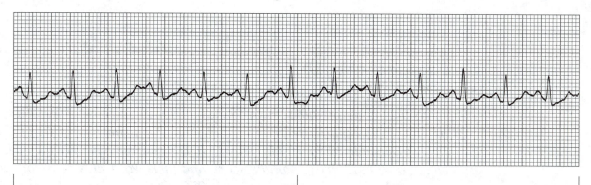

Scenario #78

Mr. Brothers, a 27-year-old male, was swimming in his Olympic swimming pool, testing his new scuba gear. His girlfriend went out to take his lunch to him and found him at the bottom of the pool. She called a neighbor to help her rescue Mr. Brothers from the pool. They call 911 to the scene, and when the paramedics arrive, bystander CPR is in progress. Aggressive advanced life support procedures are initiated; however, the patient does not respond to the resuscitative measures. The cardiac monitor initially shows the rhythm in Figure 4-78. Identify the rhythm.

Rate: _____

Rhythm: _____

P wave: _____

PRI: _____

QRS: _____

Interpretation of the rhythm strip: _____

Figure 4-78

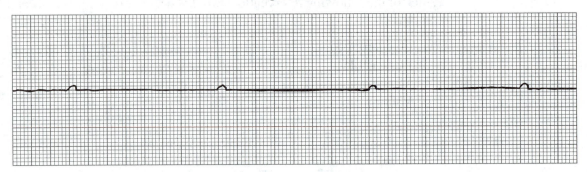

Scenario #79

Mr. Culp is a 58-year-old male who is sitting at his desk at work when he starts having palpitations. He becomes anxious and elects to call 911, as he had never experienced this type of pain. His history consists of Non-Insulin Dependent Diabetes Mellitus (NIDDM) and no other known medical conditions. EMS arrives on the scene and finds Mr. Culps conscious and oriented X3; his oxygen saturation is 97% on room air. His heart rate is irregular and he respiring at an acceptable rate. Identify Mr. Culp's ECG rhythm strip, as shown in Figure 4-79.

Rate: _____

Rhythm: _____

P wave: _____

PRI: _____

QRS: _____

Interpretation of the rhythm strip: _____

Which of the following medications would be indicated for Mr. Culp's palpitations?

- a. Viagra
- b. Nitroglycerine
- c. Morphine
- d. Oxygen

Answer: _____

Figure 4-79

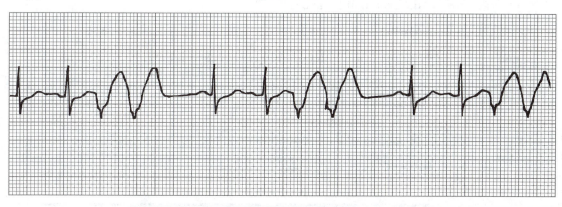

Scenario #80

Mrs. King is an 88-year-old female in the intensive care unit, receiving IV and oxygen therapy. She starts having what appears to be a grand-mal seizure. The monitor alarm starts going off, and the nurses rush in to check on the patient. They find her unresponsive with agonal respirations, and she has no pulse. She is status post acute MI. No invasive interventions were undertaken. The cardiac monitor reveals the rhythm in Figure 4-80. Identify the rhythm.

Rate: _____

Rhythm: _____

Figure 4-80

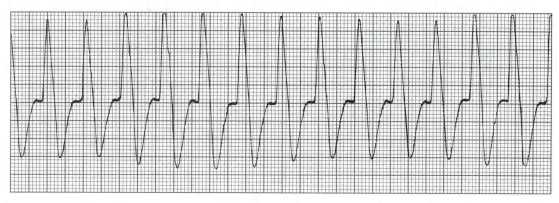

P wave: _____

PRI: _____

QRS: _____

Interpretation of the rhythm strip: _____

Since this is a witnessed arrest, the immediate intervention would be:

   a. Insertion of a demand pacemaker
   b. Immediate cardioversion
   c. Immediate defibrillation
   d. Establish IV access

Answer: _____

After the initial intervention is successful, the next step would be:

   a. Establish an IV lifeline
   b. Lidocaine 100 mg IVP
   c. Amiodarone 600 mg IV
   d. Endotracheal intubation

Answer: _____

Scenario #81

Mr. Bromburg is a 68-year-old male who awoke with chest pain. He elected to take two Nitroglycerine tablets that he had "borrowed" from his fishing buddy. When the paramedics arrive on the scene, they find Mr. Bromburg sitting in a chair in his bedroom. He is semiconscious and responds only to loud verbal stimuli. His skin is pale and cool and clammy to the touch. His oxygen saturation is 88% on room air. His heart rate is barely palpable and he respiring at a rate of 5 breaths per minute. Identify Mr. Bromburg's rhythm strip, as shown in Figure 4-81.

Figure 4-81

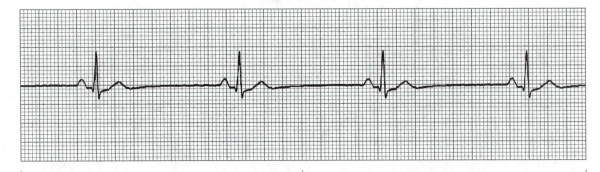

Rate: _____

Rhythm: _____

P wave: _____

PRI: _____

QRS: _____

Interpretation of the rhythm strip: _____

Which of the following medications would be indicated for Mr. Bromburg's current situation?

a. Atropine
b. Nitroglycerine
c. Morphine
d. Demerol

Answer: _____

Scenario #82

Mr. Evergreen is a 47-year-old male, who is working on a roof on the house he is currently building. He has been a carpenter for 25 years and is in excellent health, according to his coworkers. Suddenly he begins to notice some vague pains in his chest, which he, of course, decides is merely indigestion. He takes two of the Rolaids in his pocket and continues to work. Although he has experienced a few twinges of discomfort in the past 6 months, he has not mentioned this to anyone. At the end of the workday, Mr. Evergreen again begins to feel pain in his chest and thus elects to go to the emergent care clinic, which is on his route to his home. He notifies his wife to meet him at the clinic. The doctor places Mr. Evergreen on a cardiac monitor and sees the rhythm shown in Figure 4-82. Identify Mr. Evergreen's ECG rhythm strip.

Figure 4-82

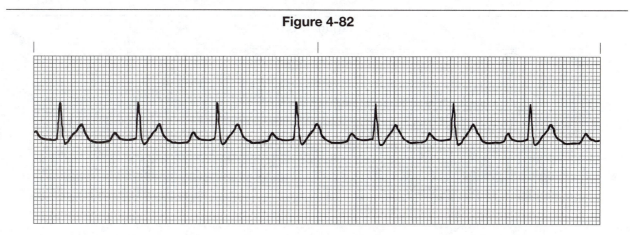

Rate: _____

Rhythm: _____

P wave: _____

PRI: _____

QRS: _____

Interpretation of the rhythm strip: _____

Scenario #83

Mrs. Burnett is a 38-year-old female who is washing her hair in the bathroom sink. She gets soap in her eyes, so she reaches for a towel and accidentally grabs her hair dryer, which has an open wire exposed. Mrs. Burnett receives an electrical shock and falls to the floor. Her 16-year-old son, who is a volunteer firefighter who has just completed a CPR course, hears the noise and runs to check on his mom. He finds her apneic and without a pulse. He shouts out to his dad to call 911 and immediately starts CPR. First responders arrive on the scene, place an AED on the patient, and it shocks her one time. CPR is continued and ALS arrives on the scene shortly afterward. They place her on a cardiac monitor and it shows the rhythm in Figure 4-83. Identify Mrs. Burnett's ECG rhythm strip.

Rate: _____

Rhythm: _____

P wave: _____

PRI: _____

QRS: _____

Interpretation of the rhythm strip: _____

Figure 4-83

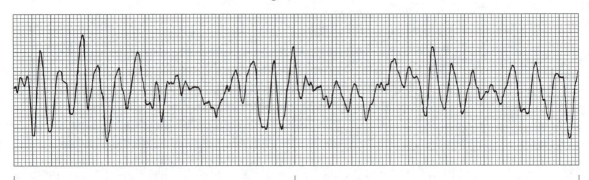

After successful intervention, which pharmacologic agent would be appropriate for Mrs. Burnett's condition?

    a. Diltiazem
    b. Amiodarone
    c. Morphine
    d. Atropine

Answer: _____

Scenario #84

Mr. Antoine is a 60-year-old male who is driving on the Interstate and begins to note palpations recurring in his chest. He has noticed this "strange feeling" off and on for about a month, but he felt he was just too busy to have them checked by a physician. He sees a sign that is announcing a new ER at the new medical center nearby and decides to have his condition checked. He takes the appropriate exit and drives to the ER. After a wait of 2 hrs, Mr. Antoine is just about to leave when he is called to the back and placed in a treatment room. He is placed on a cardiac monitor, which reveals the rhythm shown in Figure 4-84. Identify Mr. Antoine's ECG rhythm strip.

    Rate: _____

    Rhythm: _____

    P wave: _____

    PRI: _____

    QRS: _____

    Interpretation of the rhythm strip: _____

Figure 4-84

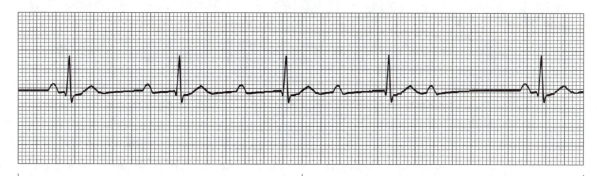

The physician who assessed Mr. Antione most likely issued him the following advice:

a. Begin taking a prescription medication called Verapamil.
b. Be a direct admit to undergo PCA.
c. Resume his previous lifestyle without adjustments.
d. Be admitted for observation.

Answer: _____

Scenario #85

Mrs. Jordan is a 76-year-old female who is going to see her physician for an annual checkup. Her physician examines her and orders an ECG. After the ECG is done, he compares it to an old ECG and notes changes. She has no significant medical history; however, she did see a convincing ad on TV for aspirin and she elected to start herself on the drug a month ago. Identify Mrs. Jordan's ECG rhythm strip, as shown in Figure 4-85.

Rate: _____

Rhythm: _____

P wave: _____

PRI: _____

QRS: _____

Interpretation of the rhythm strip: _____

Figure 4-85

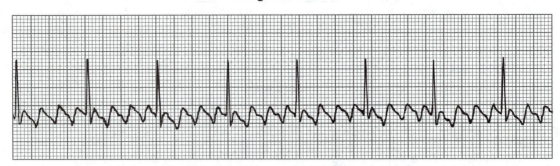

Scenario #86

Mr. Banks is a 24-year-old paramedic student, sitting at his desk in his classroom. The focus of the class today is cardiac rhythms, so Mr. Banks decides to place himself on the monitor. Much to his surprise, he notices that his rhythm is irregular. He calls his instructor over to affirm his finding. Identify Mr. Bank's ECG rhythm strip, as shown in Figure 4-86.

Rate: _____

Rhythm: _____

P wave: _____

PRI: _____

QRS: _____

Interpretation of the rhythm strip: _____

Figure 4-86

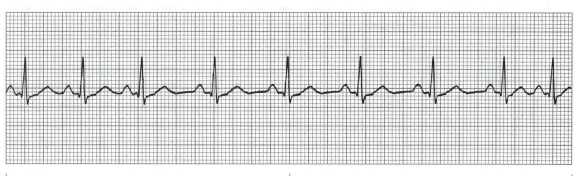

Scenario #87

Ms. Elliot is a 42-year-old career female who notices that, at times, it feels as though her heart stops and it "feels funny." Her boyfriend encourages her to get her problem checked by a doctor. She has a family history of "sudden death;" however, she has no significant medical history of which she is aware. Her family physician assesses her thoroughly, including ordering an ECG. Her rhythm strip is shown in Figure 4-87. Identify Ms. Elliot's ECG rhythm strip.

Rate: _____

Rhythm: _____

P wave: _____

PRI: _____

QRS: _____

Interpretation of the rhythm strip: _____

Figure 4-87

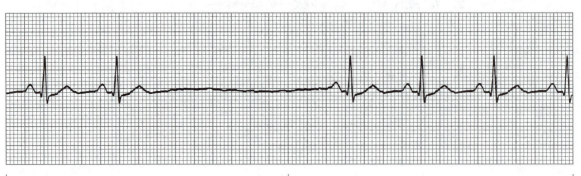

Scenario #88

Mr. Wilson is a 59-year-old male, who is sitting on a gurney in the emergency department. He presented 2 hrs ago with an irregular heartbeat. The physician has decided to admit Mr. Wilson for observation. His history consists of AHD, and he is taking an adult aspirin daily. The nurse comes in to establish an IV, and as she inserts the needle into his arm, she notes a rhythm change on the monitor. His vital signs remain stable. Identify Mr. Wilson's ECG rhythm strip, as shown in Figure 4-88.

Rate: _____

Rhythm: _____

P wave: _____

PRI: _____

QRS: _____

Interpretation of the rhythm strip: _____

Figure 4-88

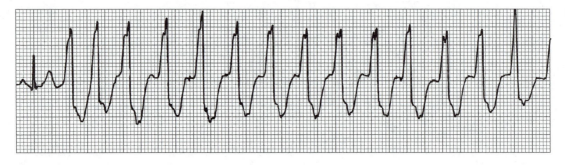

Which of the following medications would be immediately indicated for Mr. Wilson's witnessed rhythm change?

a. Atropine
b. Amiodarone
c. Procainamide
d. Cardizem

Answer: _____

Scenario #89

Mr. Lowe is a 61-year-old male, who was working in his workshop. He started having pain to his mid-chest and sat down to see if it would go away. When the pain did not subside, he went into the house and advised his wife that she needed to take him to the emergency room. She, however, decided to call 911 for an ambulance. Paramedics arrived and placed him on oxygen, which showed an oxygen saturation of 97% on a nonrebreather mask. His skin is cool, pale, and clammy. His heart rate is regular, and he respiring at an acceptable rate. Identify Mr. Lowe's ECG rhythm strip, as shown in Figure 4-89.

Rate: _____

Rhythm: _____

P wave: _____

PRI: _____

QRS: _____

Interpretation of the rhythm strip: _____

Figure 4-89

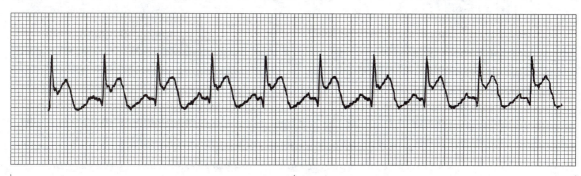

Which of the following interventions would be indicated for Mr. Lowe's condition?

a. Lidocaine after IV is established
b. Twelve-lead EKG and notify MD and if prehospital, transmit
c. External pacemaker and notify medical control
d. Cardioversion, Procainamide, Morphine sulfate

Answer: _____

Scenario #90

Mrs. Kirby is a 34-year-old female who is shopping with her sister when she begins to experience "chest pain." She is very upset by the presence of the chest pain and asks her sister to rush her to the emergency department. Her medical history is not significant. She has no known medical conditions. The ER doctor elects to do an ECG, although Mrs. Kirby has no other symptoms. Her vital signs are within normal limits. Identify Mrs. Kirby's ECG rhythm strip, as shown in Figure 4-90.

Rate: _____

Rhythm: _____

P wave: _____

PRI: _____

QRS: _____

Interpretation of the rhythm strip: _____

Figure 4-90

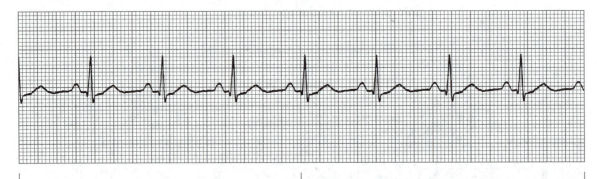

Scenario #91

Mr. Lindsey is a 50-year-old male who arrived home from his office at 6 p.m. His wife reports that he was about to cut grass in their yard when he clutched his chest and complained of chest pain. She reports that he then "fell out," and she could not get him to answer her questions. She immediately phones 911, where the emergency dispatcher begins to coach her in CPR techniques. The couple's neighbor is a firefighter and has an AED in his truck. He defibrillates the patient once with his AED and is now performing CPR. The patient's medical history is not significant and he has no known medical conditions. The patient's vital signs are absent. Identify Mr. Lindsey's ECG rhythm strip, as shown in Figure 4-91.

Rate: _____

Rhythm: _____

P wave: _____

PRI: _____

QRS: _____

Interpretation of the rhythm strip: _____

You realize this patient is experiencing:

a. AV dissociation
b. Pulseless electrical activity
c. Congestive heart failure
d. Aortic aneurysm rupture

Answer: _____

Figure 4-91

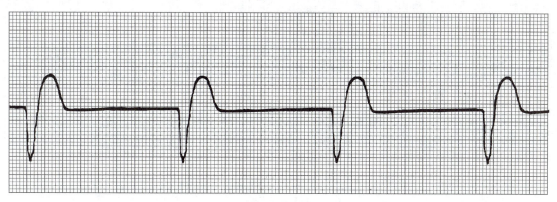

Scenario #92

You and your partner are dispatched to the scene of an apartment complex, where you find a 30-year-old female who is very agitated and is pacing the floor and wringing her hands. She is very upset by the presence of chest pain and reports that she "took a hit of crack cocaine" because she thought it would help her pain. After much coercion, she agrees to treatment. Her medical history is not significant, except for the use of cocaine "on occasion." The ER medical direction doctor instructs you to transport the patient to the ER after obtaining an ECG. Her vital signs are: blood pressure, 200/100; heart rate, 140; respiration of 36 breaths per minute. Identify the patient's ECG rhythm strip, as shown in Figure 4-92.

Rate: _____

Rhythm: _____

P wave: _____

PRI: _____

QRS: _____

Interpretation of the rhythm strip: _____

Medical conditions that occur secondary to cocaine use include:

  a. Lethargy and normotension
  b. Decreased myocardial consumption
  c. Myocardial ischemia
  d. Deep-vein thrombosis

Answer: _____

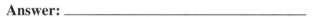

Figure 4-92

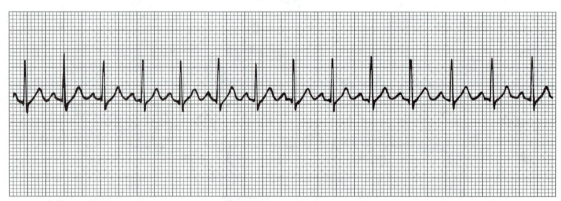

Scenario #93

Mr. Johnson is a 60-year-old male who has experienced multiple medical issues with his health in the past 5 years, based on a medical history offered by his wife. She calls the emergency department while driving to the hospital to bring her husband. Prior to the past 5 years, Mr. Johnson's medical history is not significant. He began to complain with "bad indigestion" approximately 1 hr earlier. Upon arrival at the ER, the doctor elects to do an ECG. His vital signs are: blood pressure, 130/80; heart rate, 98; and respiration rate of 24 breaths per minute. The doctor instructs the nurse to administer three baby aspirin, followed by sublingual nitroglycerin (0.4 mg) for his chest pain. Identify Mr. Johnson's ECG rhythm strip, as shown in Figure 4-93.

Rate: _____

Rhythm: _____

P wave: _____

PRI: _____

QRS: _____

Interpretation of the rhythm strip: _____

The screening methodology most frequently utilized in the prehospital arena, as well as in the emergency department, to evaluate patients who present with chest pain is the:

   a. Pulse oximeter
   b. Sphygmomanometer
   c. Electrocardiogram
   d. Initiation of intravenous fluids

Answer: _____

Figure 4-93

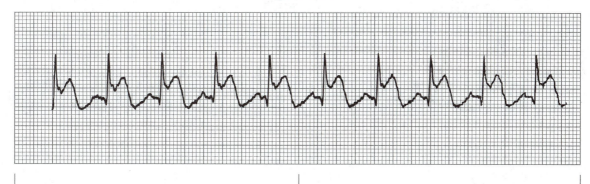

Scenario #94

Mr. Henderson is a 66-year-old male who is attending a family reunion with his wife when he begins to experience "chest pain." He is alert and communicative with you and your partner when you enter the Fellowship Hall in the church where the reunion is being held. He began to feel dizzy, and his family encourages him to lie down. Prior to transporting the patient to the emergency department, you complete an assessment and note that his blood pressure is 144/96, his heart rate is 58 and irregular, and he is respiring at a rate of 24 breaths per minute. His medical history reveals only infrequent episodes of moderate hypertension. The patient is placed on a cardiac monitor, which reveals the rhythm strip shown in Figure 4-94.

Rate: _____

Rhythm: _____

P wave: _____

PRI: _____

QRS: _____

Interpretation of the rhythm strip: _____

Your initial treatment should be to:

a. Initiate IV lifeline
b. Intubate the patient
c. Institute 100% oxygen via NRB
d. Begin a Lidocaine drip via IVPB

Answer: _____

Figure 4-94

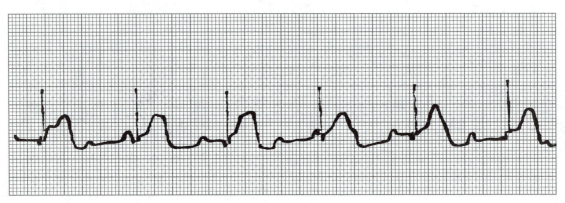

Scenario #95

Mrs. Lee is a 48-year-old female who is busy in her kitchen preparing for the holiday season, and she has been cooking since about 7 a.m. It is now 1 p.m. and she notes that she is feeling tired and has some mild chest pain. She is very upset by the presence of the chest pain and asks her daughter to take her to her doctor's office. She has no significant medical history. Her only known allergy is to penicillin. Her doctor elects to do an ECG. Her vital signs are within normal limits. Identify Mrs. Lee's ECG rhythm strip, as shown in Figure 4-95.

Rate: _____

Rhythm: _____

P wave: _____

PRI: _____

QRS: _____

Interpretation of the rhythm strip: _____

Figure 4-95

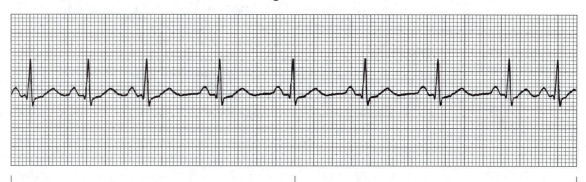

Scenario #96

Mr. McDaniel is a 61-year-old male who is enjoying a round of golf with his son when he begins to experience chest pain. He holds his chest and falls to the ground. His son calls 911 on his cell phone, and begins CPR on his father. There is no AED at the clubhouse, so his son continues CPR until the paramedics arrive. They immediately begin ACLS protocols on Mr. McDaniel. His ECG rhythm strip is shown in Figure 4-96.

Rate: _____

Rhythm: _____

Figure 4-96

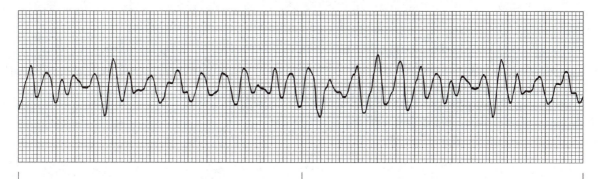

P wave: _____

PRI: _____

QRS: _____

Interpretation of the rhythm strip: _____

Immediately after the initial defibrillation is delivered at 200 biphasic, the next appropriate action would be:

a. Administer 300 mg of sodium bicarbonate
b. Initiate intravenous access bilaterally
c. Deliver five cycles of CPR prior to rhythm interpretation
d. Deliver three sets of "stacked" shocks to the patient

Answer: _____

Scenario #97

Mr. Jensen is a 60-year-old male who is a patient in the progressive care unit at your hospital. He presses his call button, and, when you check on him, he explains that he is experiencing chest pain. He appears uncomfortable and you note that he is diaphoretic. You immediately check his vital signs and note the following: blood pressure, 134/86; heart rate,120 BPM; respirations, 18 per minute. His oxygen saturation is 95% on room air. The attending doctor asks you to do a 12-lead ECG. Identify Mr. Jensen's ECG rhythm strip, as shown in Figure 4-97.

Rate: _____

Rhythm: _____

P wave: _____

Figure 4-97

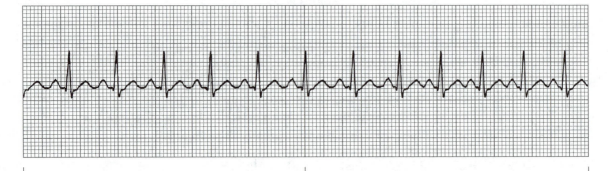

PRI: _____

QRS: _____

Interpretation of the rhythm strip: _____

Scenario #98

Mrs. Patterson is a 74-year-old female who suddenly collapses at home. Her sister had joined her for lunch and subsequently calls 911. You and your crew arrived within 4 min and find Mrs. Patterson to be without pulse and apneic. You begin CPR and attach the cardiac monitor. Her sister states that the patient is "very healthy" and has no known medical conditions. Identify Mrs. Patterson's ECG rhythm strip, as shown in Figure 4-98.

Rate: _____

Rhythm: _____

P wave: _____

PRI: _____

QRS: _____

Interpretation of the rhythm strip: _____

What is the more appropriate next step?

    a. Deliver a precordial thump and observe the patient's rhythm.
    b. Defibrillate immediately and continue CPR.
    c. Establish venous access and defibrillate.
    d. Continue 2 min of CPR, and recheck the rhythm.

Answer: _____

Figure 4-98

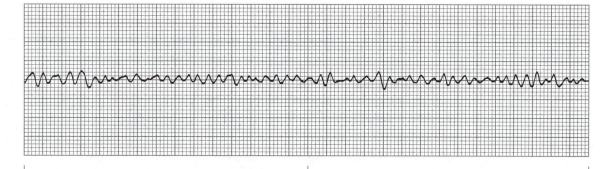

Scenario #99

Mrs. Stewart has just experienced a panic attack, according to her husband, who answers the door as you respond to a 911 call and arrive on the scene. He relates that she had an argument with her friend and became very upset. He noticed that she began to hyperventilate and became very upset, so he called for help. The patient breathlessly tells you that her heart is "beating funny." With the exception of a respiratory rate of 32, her vital signs are within normal limits when you check. Identify Mrs. Stewart's ECG rhythm strip, as shown in Figure 4-99.

Rate: _____

Rhythm: _____

P wave: _____

PRI: _____

QRS: _____

Interpretation of the rhythm strip: _____

Figure 4-99

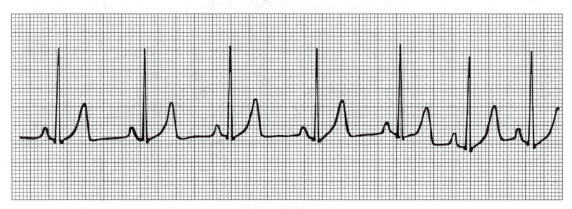

Scenario #100

Mrs. Morrison is a 37-year-old female who is visiting her family physician with complaints of "extreme fatigue." She has no other specific complaints. Her physician elects to do a number of lab tests as well as obtain an ECG. Her medical history is not significant. She has no known medical conditions. Her vital signs are within normal limits. Identify Mrs. Morrison's ECG rhythm strip, as shown in Figure 4-100.

Rate: _____

Rhythm: _____

P wave: _____

PRI: _____

QRS: _____

Interpretation of the rhythm strip: _____

Figure 4-100

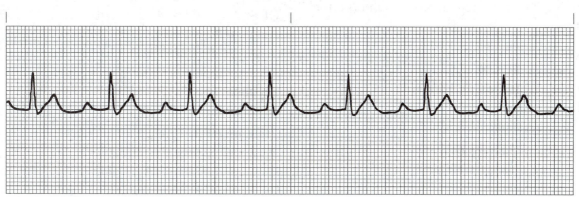

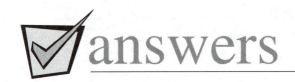
answers

Scenario #1

Utilizing the five-step approach, interpret the rhythm.

Rate: 70
Rhythm: Regular
P wave: Present and upright
PRI: 0.16
QRS: 0.06

What is your Interpretation of this patient's rhythm strip? Normal sinus rhythm

Scenario #2

Rate: 40
Rhythm: Regular
P wave: Present and upright
PRI: 0.16
QRS: 0.04

Interpretation of the rhythm strip: Sinus bradycardia

Scenario #3

Rate: 120
Rhythm: Regular
P wave: Present and upright
PRI: 0.16
QRS: 0.06

Interpretation of the rhythm strip: Sinus tachycardia

Scenario #4

Rate: 60
Rhythm: Irregular

P wave: Present and upright
PRI: 0.16
QRS: 0.04

Interpretation of the rhythm strip: Sinus rhythm with sinus arrest

Scenario #5

Rate: 90
Rhythm: Irregular
P wave: Indistinguishable
PRI: Indistinguishable
QRS: 0.04

Interpretation of the rhythm strip: Atrial fibrillation

Answer to question: c

Scenario #6

Rate: 50
Rhythm: Regular
P wave: Inverted
PRI: 0.10
QRS: 0.04

Interpretation of the rhythm strip: Junctional rhythm

Scenario #7

Rate: 80
Rhythm: Irregular
P wave: Present and upright
PRI: 0.16
QRS: 0.08

Interpretation of the rhythm strip: Sinus rhythm with unifocal PVCs

Scenario #8

Rate:	70
Rhythm:	Irregular
P wave:	Present and upright
PRI:	0.16
QRS:	0.04

Interpretation of the rhythm strip: Sinus rhythm with multifocal PVCs, bigeminy

Answer to question: a

Scenario #9

Rate:	> 200
Rhythm:	Irregular
P wave:	Absent
PRI:	Absent
QRS:	> 0.12

Interpretation of the rhythm strip: Course ventricular fibrillation

Scenario #10

Rate:	0
Rhythm:	0
P wave:	0
PRI:	0
QRS:	0

Interpretation of the rhythm strip: Asystole

Answer to question: a

Scenario #11

Rate:	70
Rhythm:	Regular
P wave:	Present and upright
PRI:	0.24
QRS:	0.08

Interpretation of the rhythm strip: Sinus rhythm with first-degree block

Scenario #12

Rate:	> 200
Rhythm:	Irregular

P wave:	Absent
PRI:	Absent
QRS:	> 0.12

Interpretation of the rhythm strip: Course Ventricular fibrillation

Scenario #13

Rate:	20
Rhythm:	Regular
P wave:	Present and upright
PRI:	Variable
QRS:	> 0.12

Interpretation of the rhythm strip: Third-degree block

Scenario #14

Rate:	140
Rhythm:	Regular
P wave:	Absent
PRI:	Absent
QRS:	0.28

Interpretation of the rhythm strip: Ventricular tachycardia

Answer to question: c

Scenario #15

Rate:	60
Rhythm:	Regular
P wave:	Present and upright
PRI:	0.18
QRS:	0.06

Interpretation of the rhythm strip: Second-degree block type II (Mobitz II) with inverted T wave

Scenario #16

Rate:	90
Rhythm:	Irregular
P wave:	Present and upright
PRI:	0.16
QRS:	0.04

Interpretation of the rhythm strip: Sinus dysrhythmia

Scenario #17

Rate: 80
Rhythm: Regular
P wave: a (f waves)
PRI: Absent
QRS: 0.04

Interpretation of the rhythm strip: Atrial flutter

Scenario #18

Rate: 260
Rhythm: Regular
P wave: Indistinguishable
PRI: Indistinguishable
QRS: 0.04

Interpretation of the rhythm strip: Supraventricular tachycardia

Scenario #19

Rate: 70
Rhythm: Regular
P wave: Absent
PRI: Absent
QRS: 0.06

Interpretation of the rhythm strip: Accelerated junctional rhythm

Scenario #20

Rate: > 200
Rhythm: Irregular
P wave: Absent
PRI: Absent
QRS: Absent

Interpretation of the rhythm strip: Ventricular fibrillation

Scenario #21

Rate: 30
Rhythm: Regular
P wave: Present and upright
PRI: Variable
QRS: 0.12

Interpretation of the rhythm strip: Third-degree block

Scenario #22

Rate: 80
Rhythm: Regular
P wave: Present and upright
PRI: 0.12
QRS: 0.10

Interpretation of the rhythm strip: Atrial paced rhythm with ST elevation

Scenario #23

Rate: > 200
Rhythm: Irregular
P wave: Present and upright in first six complexes
PRI: 0.16 in first six complexes
QRS: 0.08 in first six complexes

Interpretation of the rhythm strip: Normal sinus rhythm going in to V tach and v fib

Answer to question: b

Scenario #24

Rate: Undetermined
Rhythm: Irregular
P wave: Absent
PRI: Absent
QRS: Absent

Interpretation of the rhythm strip: Ventricular fibrillation with conversion

Answer to question: d

Scenario #25

Rate: 70
Rhythm: Regular
P wave: Present and upright
PRI: 0.22
QRS: 0.08

Interpretation of the rhythm strip: PEA. Underlying rhythm is first-degree heart block

Answer to question: a

Scenario #26

Rate: 70
Rhythm: Irregular
P wave: Indistinguishable
PRI: Indistinguishable
QRS: 0.08

Interpretation of the rhythm strip: A fib with ST elevation

Answer to question: a

Scenario #27

Rate: 80
Rhythm: Regular
P wave: Present and upright
PRI: 0.20
QRS: 0.04

Interpretation of the rhythm strip: Normal sinus rhythm

Scenario #28

Rate: 110
Rhythm: Regular
P wave: Present and upright
PRI: 0.16
QRS: 0.08

Interpretation of the rhythm strip: Sinus tachycardia

Scenario #29

Rate: 150
Rhythm: Regular
P wave: Absent
PRI: Absent
QRS: > 0.12

Interpretation of the rhythm strip: Ventricular tachycardia

Answer to question: a

Scenario #30

Rate: 30
Rhythm: Regular
P wave: Absent
PRI: 0.16
QRS: 0.04

Interpretation of the rhythm strip: Junctional rhythm

Answer to question 1: d

Answer to question 2: c

Scenario #31

Rate: 50
Rhythm: Irregular
P wave: Present and upright
PRI: 0.26
QRS: 0.08

Interpretation of the rhythm strip: Second-degree AV type II block, variable 2:1 and 3:1 ratios

Scenario #32

Rate: 60
Rhythm: Regular
P wave: Present and upright
PRI: 0.16
QRS: 0.04

Interpretation of the rhythm strip: Normal sinus rhythm with ST elevation

Scenario #33

Rate: 140
Rhythm: Regular
P wave: Present and upright
PRI: 0.16
QRS: 0.04

Interpretation of the rhythm strip: Sinus tachycardia

Answer to question 1: b

Answer to question 2: d

Scenario #34

Rate: 70
Rhythm: Irregular
P wave: Present and upright
PRI: 0.20
QRS: 0.04

Interpretation of the rhythm strip: Sinus Rhythm with 5th complex pvc, consider R on T

Answer to question: a

Scenario #35

Rate: 40
Rhythm: Irregular
P wave: Present and upright
PRI: 0.16
QRS: 0.04

Interpretation of the rhythm strip: Second-degree block type II, 2:1 ratio

Answer to question: c

Scenario #36

Rate: 80
Rhythm: Regular
P wave: Present and upright
PRI: 0.16
QRS: 0.06

Interpretation of the rhythm strip: Normal sinus rhythm

Scenario #37

Rate: 90
Rhythm: Irregular
P wave: Indistinguishable
PRI: Indistinguishable
QRS: 0.06

Interpretation of the rhythm strip: Atrial fibrillation

Scenario #38

Rate: 40
Rhythm: Regular

P wave: Present and upright
PRI: 0.16
QRS: 0.04

Interpretation of the rhythm strip: Sinus bradycardia

Answer to question: c

Scenario #39

Rate: Indistinguishable
Rhythm: Indistinguishable
P wave: Indistinguishable
PRI: Indistinguishable
QRS: Indistinguishable

Interpretation of the rhythm strip: Coarse ventricular fibrillation

Answer to question: b

Scenario #40

Rate: 170
Rhythm: Regular
P wave: Absent
PRI: Absent
QRS: > 0.12

Interpretation of the rhythm strip: Ventricular tachycardia

Answer to question: b

Scenario #41

Rate: 100
Rhythm: Regular
P wave: Present and upright
PRI: 0.16
QRS: 0.08

Interpretation of the rhythm strip: Sinus rachycardia with ST segment elevation

Answer to question: c

Scenario #42

Rate: 70
Rhythm: Irregular

P wave: Present and upright
PRI: Variable
QRS: 0.08

Interpretation of the rhythm strip: Second-degree block type I

Scenario #43

Rate: 20
Rhythm: Regular
P wave: Present and upright
PRI: Variable
QRS: 0.12

Interpretation of the rhythm strip: Third-degree heart block

Answer to question: d

Scenario #44

Rate: 80
Rhythm: Irregular
P wave: Present and upright
PRI: 0.18
QRS: 0.08

Interpretation of the rhythm strip: Sinus rhythm with unifocal pvc (bigeminy)

Scenario #45

Rate: 50
Rhythm: Regular
P wave: Inverted
PRI: 0.12
QRS: 0.04

Interpretation of the rhythm strip: Junctional escape rhythm

Scenario #46

Rate: 40
Rhythm: Regular
P wave: Varies
PRI: Varies
QRS: 0.12

Interpretation of the rhythm strip: Malfunctioning pacemaker and third-degree block

Scenario #47

Rate: 50
Rhythm: Irregularly irregular
P wave: Indistinguishable
PRI: Indistinguishable
QRS: 0.06

Interpretation of the rhythm strip: Atrial fibrillation

Scenario #48

Rate: 210
Rhythm: Regular
P wave: Indistinguishable
PRI: Indistinguishable
QRS: 0.06

Interpretation of the rhythm strip: Supraventricular tachycardia

Answer to question: c

Scenario #49

Rate: Indistinguishable
Rhythm: Indistinguishable
P wave: Indistinguishable
PRI: Indistinguishable
QRS: Indistinguishable

Interpretation of the rhythm strip: Ventricular asystole

Scenario #50

Rate: 60
Rhythm: Irregular
P wave: Present and upright
PRI: Variable
QRS: 0.04

Interpretation of the rhythm strip: Second-degree block Mobitz type I

Scenario #51

Rate:	40
Rhythm:	Regular
P wave:	Present upright
PRI:	0.16
QRS:	0.08

Interpretation of the rhythm strip: Sinus bradycardia

Scenario #52

Rate:	80
Rhythm:	Irregular
P wave:	Present and upright
PRI:	0.12
QRS:	0.04

Interpretation of the rhythm strip: Sinus dysrhythmia

Scenario #53

Rate:	120
Rhythm:	Regular
P wave:	Present and upright
PRI:	0.16
QRS:	0.04

Interpretation of the rhythm strip: Sinus tachycardia

Scenario #54

Rate:	60
Rhythm:	Irregular
P wave:	Present and upright
PRI:	0.16
QRS:	0.04

Interpretation of the rhythm strip: Sinus arrest

Scenario #55

Rate:	90
Rhythm:	Irregular
P wave:	Not present, fib waves
PRI:	Not present
QRS:	0.04

Interpretation of the rhythm strip: Atrial fibrillation

Answer to question: c

Scenario #56

Rate:	50
Rhythm:	Regular
P wave:	Inverted
PRI:	0.12
QRS:	0.04

Interpretation of the rhythm strip: Junctional escape rhythm

Scenario #57

Rate:	80
Rhythm:	Irregular
P wave:	Present and upright
PRI:	0.18
QRS:	0.08

Interpretation of the rhythm strip: Sinus rhythm with ST elevation and unifocal PVCs

Scenario #58

Rate:	70
Rhythm:	Irregular
P wave:	Present and upright
PRI:	0.16
QRS:	0.04

Interpretation of the rhythm strip: Sinus rhythm with multifocal bigeminy PVCs

Answer to question: b

Scenario #59

Rate:	Undetermined
Rhythm:	Irregular
P wave:	No P waves noted
PRI:	No PRI
QRS:	Wide complex

Interpretation of the rhythm strip: Torsades de pointes

Scenario #60

Rate:	Undetermined
Rhythm:	Irregular

P wave: None
PRI: None
QRS: None

Interpretation of the rhythm strip: Coarse V fib

Scenario #61

Rate: 70
Rhythm: Regular
P wave: Present and upright
PRI: 0.24
QRS: 0.04

Interpretation of the rhythm strip: sinus rhythm with first-degree heart block

Scenario #62

Rate: None
Rhythm: None
P wave: None
PRI: None
QRS: None

Interpretation of the rhythm strip: Asystole

Scenario #63

Rate: 188
Rhythm: Regular
P wave: None
PRI: None
QRS: Wide complex

Interpretation of the rhythm strip: Ventricular tachycardia

Answer to question 1: b

Answer to question 2: b

Scenario #64

Rate: 60
Rhythm: Regular
P wave: Present
PRI: None
QRS: 0.08

Interpretation of the rhythm strip: Third-degree block

Scenario #65

Rate: 70
Rhythm: Irregular
P wave: Present and upright
PRI: 0.12
QRS: 0.04

Interpretation of the rhythm strip: Sinus rhythm with bigeminy; unifocal PVCs

Scenario #66

Rate: 40
Rhythm: Regular
P wave: Present and upright
PRI: 0.24
QRS: 0.12

Interpretation of the rhythm strip: Second-degree block type II with 2:1 conduction

Scenario #67

Rate: 170
Rhythm: Regular
P wave: Not present
PRI: Not present
QRS: > 0.12

Interpretation of the rhythm strip: Ventricular tachycardia

Answer to question: c

Scenario #68

Rate: 90
Rhythm: Irregular
P wave: Not present
PRI: Not present
QRS: 0.04

Interpretation of the rhythm strip: Atrial fibrillation

Scenario #69

Rate: 80
Rhythm: Regular
P wave: Variable

PRI: Variable
QRS: 0.08

Interpretation of the rhythm strip: Third-degree heart block

Scenario #70

Rate: 70
Rhythm: Regular
P wave: Flutter waves
PRI: Indistinguishable
QRS: 0.04

Interpretation of the rhythm strip: Atrial flutter

Scenario #71

Rate: 118
Rhythm: Regular
P wave: Present and upright
PRI: 0.12
QRS: 0.04

Interpretation of the rhythm strip: Sinus tachycardia

Answer to question: b

Scenario #72

Rate: 40
Rhythm: Regular
P wave: Present and upright
PRI: 0.24
QRS: 0.08

Interpretation of the rhythm strip: Second-degree heart block; 2:1 block

Answer to question: b

Scenario #73

Rate: 30
Rhythm: Regular
P wave: Absent
PRI: Absent
QRS: 0.06

Interpretation of the rhythm strip: Junctional bradycardia

Answer to question: c

Scenario #74

Rate: 190
Rhythm: Regular
P wave: Indistinguishable
PRI: Indistinguishable
QRS: 0.04

Interpretation of the rhythm strip: Supraventricular tachycardia

Answer to question: a

Scenario #75

Rate: 100
Rhythm: Regular
P wave: Indistinguishable
PRI: Indistinguishable
QRS: 0.12

Interpretation of the rhythm strip: Accelerated Idioventricular rhythm

Answer to question: b

Scenario #76

Rate: 60
Rhythm: Irregular
P wave: Present and upright
PRI: 0.16
QRS: 0.08

Interpretation of the rhythm strip: Ventricular trigeminy

Answer to question: b

Scenario #77

Rate: 130
Rhythm: Irregular
P wave: Present and upright
PRI: 0.12
QRS: 0.04

Interpretation of the rhythm strip: Sinus tachycardia with occasional PACs

Answer to question: c

Scenario #78

Rate: 0
Rhythm: Regular
P wave: Present and upright
PRI: Absent
QRS: Absent

Interpretation of the rhythm strip: Ventricular standstill

Scenario #79

Rate: 120
Rhythm: Irregular
P wave: Present and upright
PRI: 0.16
QRS: 0.04

Interpretation of the rhythm strip: Sinus rhythm with couplet PVCs

Answer to question: d

Scenario #80

Rate: 130
Rhythm: Regular
P wave: Indistinguishable
PRI: Absent
QRS: 0.28

Interpretation of the rhythm strip: Ventricular tachycardia

Answer to question 1: c

Answer to question 2: b

Scenario #81

Rate: 40
Rhythm: Regular
P wave: Present and upright
PRI: 0.16
QRS: 0.04

Interpretation of the rhythm strip: Sinus bradycardia

Answer to question: a

Scenario #82

Rate: 70
Rhythm: Regular
P wave: Present and upright
PRI: 0.24
QRS: 0.08

Interpretation of the rhythm strip: First-degree heart block

Scenario #83

Rate: Indistinguishable
Rhythm: Irregular
P wave: Absent
PRI: Absent
QRS: Indistinguishable

Interpretation of the rhythm strip: Coarse ventricular fibrillation

Answer to question: b

Scenario #84

Rate: 50
Rhythm: Irregular
P wave: Present and upright
PRI: Increasing in length with consecutive beats
QRS: 0.04

Interpretation of the rhythm strip: Mobitz type I; second-degree heart block

Answer to question: d

Scenario #85

Rate: 80
Rhythm: Regular
P wave: Flutter waves
PRI: Indistinguishable
QRS: 0.04

Interpretation of the rhythm strip: Atrial flutter

Scenario #86

Rate: 90
Rhythm: Irregular

P wave: Present and upright
PRI: 0.16
QRS: 0.04

Interpretation of the rhythm strip: Sinus dysrhythmia

Scenario #87

Rate: 60
Rhythm: Irregular
P wave: Present and upright
PRI: 0.16
QRS: 0.04

Interpretation of the rhythm strip: Sinus arrest

Scenario #88

Rate: 150
Rhythm: Irregular
P wave: Present and upright in the first complex; otherwise absent
PRI: 0.12 in first complex only; otherwise absent
QRS: 0.06 in first complex only; in other complexes, > 1.2 seconds

Interpretation of the rhythm strip: Paroxysmal ventricular tachycardia

Answer to question: b

Scenario #89

Rate: 100
Rhythm: Regular
P wave: Present and upright
PRI: 0.16
QRS: 0.08

Interpretation of the rhythm strip: Sinus rhythm with ST segment elevation

Answer to question: b

Scenario #90

Rate: 70
Rhythm: Regular
P wave: Present and upright

PRI: 0.16
QRS: 0.04

Interpretation of the rhythm strip: Normal sinus rhythm

Scenario #91

Rate: 40
Rhythm: Regular
P wave: Absent
PRI: Absent
QRS: 0.16

Interpretation of the rhythm strip: Idioventricular rhythm

Answer to question: b

Scenario #92

Rate: 136
Rhythm: Regular
P wave: Present and upright
PRI: 0.18
QRS: 0.06

Interpretation of the rhythm strip: Sinus tachycardia

Answer to question: c

Scenario #93

Rate: 100
Rhythm: Regular
P wave: Present and upright
PRI: 0.16
QRS: 0.08

Interpretation of the rhythm strip: Sinus tachycardia with ST elevation

Answer to question: c

Scenario #94

Rate: 60
Rhythm: Regular
P wave: Present and upright
PRI: Varies
QRS: 0.08

Interpretation of the rhythm strip: Third-degree block

Answer to question: c

Scenario #95

Rate: 90
Rhythm: Irregular
P wave: Present and upright
PRI: 0.16
QRS: 0.04

Interpretation of the rhythm strip: Sinus dysrhythmia

Scenario #96

Rate: Indistinguishable
Rhythm: Indistinguishable
P wave: Absent
PRI: Absent
QRS: Absent

Interpretation of the rhythm strip: Coarse ventricular fibrillation

Answer to question: c

Scenario #97

Rate: 120
Rhythm: Regular
P wave: Present and upright
PRI: 0.16
QRS: 0.04

Interpretation of the rhythm strip: Sinus tachycardia rhythm

Scenario #98

Rate: Indistinguishable
Rhythm: Indistinguishable
P wave: Absent
PRI: Absent
QRS: Absent

Interpretation of the rhythm strip: Fine ventricular fibrillation

Answer to question: b

Scenario #99

Rate: 70
Rhythm: Regular
P wave: Present and upright
PRI: 0.16
QRS: 0.04

Interpretation of the rhythm strip: Sinus dysrhythmia

Scenario #100

Rate: 70
Rhythm: Regular
P wave: Present and upright
PRI: 0.24
QRS: 0.04

Interpretation of the rhythm strip: First-degree heart block

CHAPTER
5
More Review Rhythm Strips

This chapter is included in order to provide review strips that will reinforce your knowledge of ECG interpretation. We encourage you to apply the five-step approach to interpret each of the following strips.

When you have finished with your interpretation of these 400 strips, you should then *turn to the back of the chapter to check your answers with the answers provided in this appendix*. It should be assumed that all strips are 6-second strips unless otherwise indicated. Some rhythm strips are shown with more than one lead for the sake of clarity.

Now go ahead and utilize your ECG interpretation skills and enjoy this challenge! We wish you Happy Reviewing!

Brenda and Mike

Note:

Rate and rhythm refer to ventricular rate and rhythm, unless otherwise noted.

A denotes Absent.

V denotes Variable.

I denotes Indiscernible or Indistinguishable.

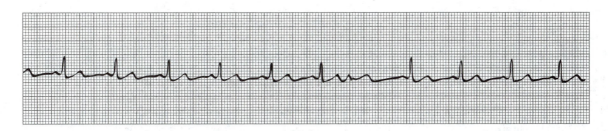

1. Rate: _____
   Rhythm: _____
   P wave: _____
   PRI: _____
   QRS: _____

   Interpretation: _____

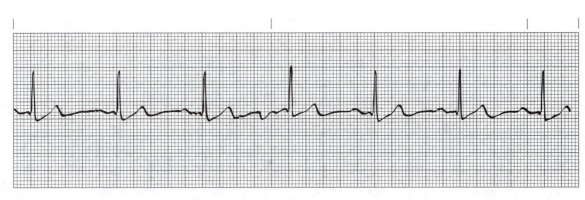

2. Rate: _____
   Rhythm: _____
   P wave: _____
   PRI: _____
   QRS: _____

   Interpretation: _____

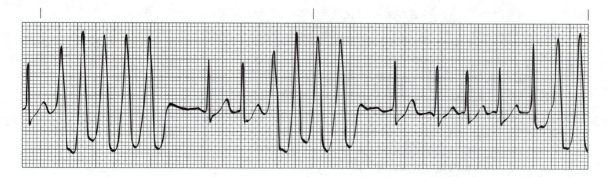

3. Rate: _____

   Rhythm: _____

   P wave: _____

   PRI: _____

   QRS: _____

   Interpretation: _____

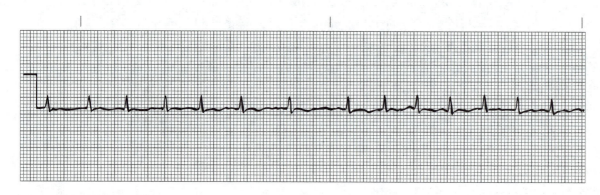

4. Rate: _____

   Rhythm: _____

   P wave: _____

   PRI: _____

   QRS: _____

   Interpretation: _____

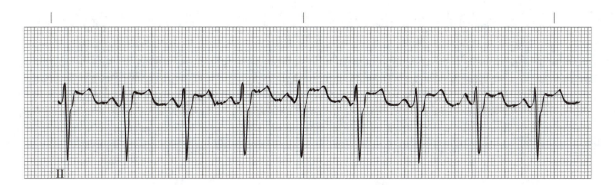

5. Rate: _____

   Rhythm: _____

   P wave: _____

   PRI: _____

   QRS: _____

   Interpretation: _____

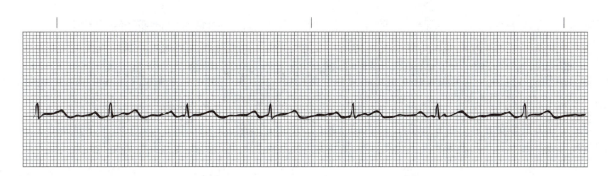

6. Rate: _____

   Rhythm: _____

   P wave: _____

   PRI: _____

   QRS: _____

   Interpretation: _____

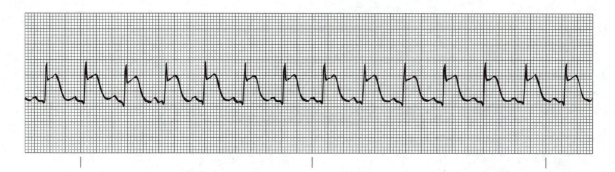

7. Rate: _____

Rhythm: _____

P wave: _____

PRI: _____

QRS: _____

Interpretation: _____

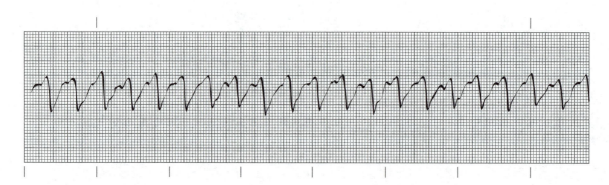

8. Rate: _____

Rhythm: _____

P waves: _____

PRI: _____

QRS: _____

Interpretation: _____

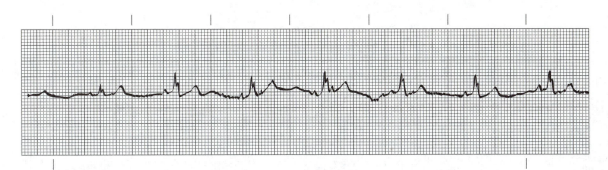

9. Rate: _____
   Rhythm: _____
   P wave: _____
   PRI: _____
   QRS: _____

   Interpretation: _____

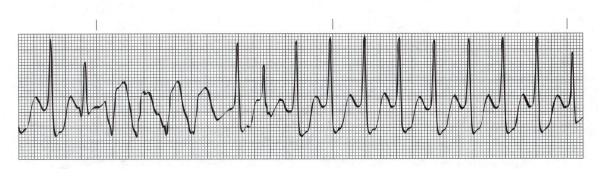

10. Rate: _____
    Rhythm: _____
    P wave: _____
    PRI: _____
    QRS: _____

    Interpretation: _____

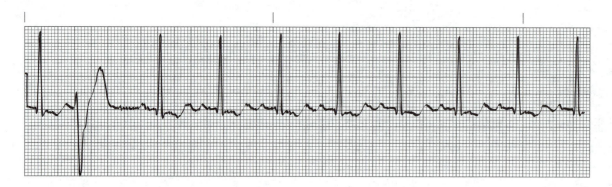

11. Rate: _____

    Rhythm: _____

    P wave: _____

    PRI: _____

    QRS: _____

    Interpretation: _____

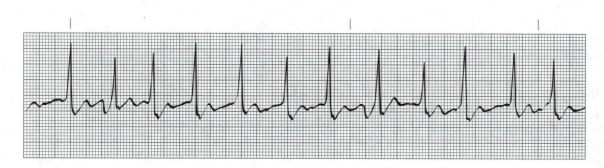

12. Rate: _____

    Rhythm: _____

    P wave: _____

    PRI: _____

    QRS: _____

    Interpretation: _____

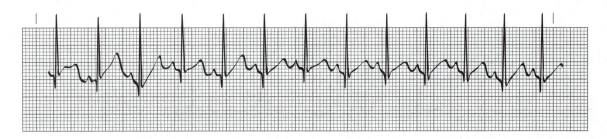

13. Rate: _____

    Rhythm: _____

    P wave: _____

    PRI: _____

    QRS: _____

    Interpretation: _____

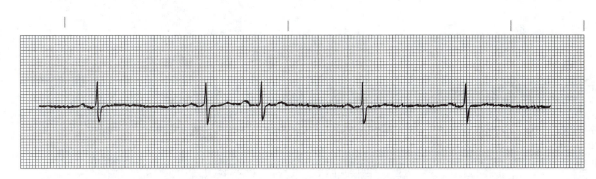

14. Rate: _____

    Rhythm: _____

    P wave: _____

    PRI: _____

    QRS: _____

    Interpretation: _____

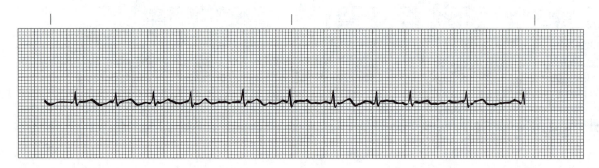

15. Rate: _____

    Rhythm: _____

    P waves: _____

    PRI: _____

    QRS: _____

    Interpretation: _____

16. Rate: _____

    Rhythm: _____

    P wave: _____

    PRI: _____

    QRS: _____

    Interpretation: _____

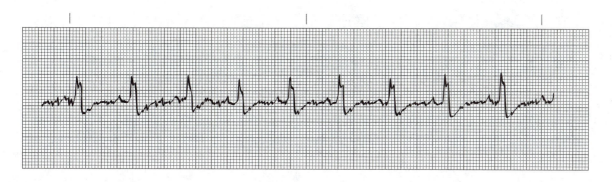

17. Rate: _____

    Rhythm: _____

    P wave: _____

    PRI: _____

    QRS: _____

    Interpretation: _____

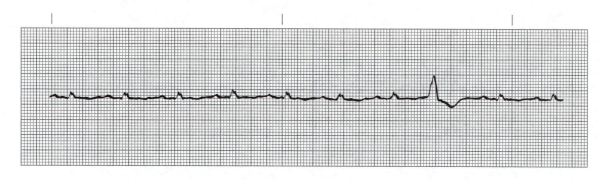

18. Rate: _____

    Rhythm: _____

    P wave: _____

    PRI: _____

    QRS: _____

    Interpretation: _____

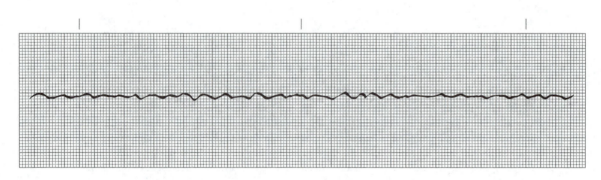

19. Rate: _____
    Rhythm: _____
    P wave: _____
    PRI: _____
    QRS: _____

    Interpretation: _____

20. Rate: _____
    Rhythm: _____
    P wave: _____
    PRI: _____
    QRS: _____

    Interpretation: _____

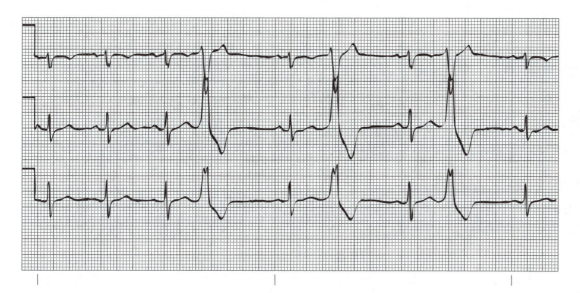

21. Rate: _____

    Rhythm: _____

    P wave: _____

    PRI: _____

    QRS: _____

    Interpretation: _____

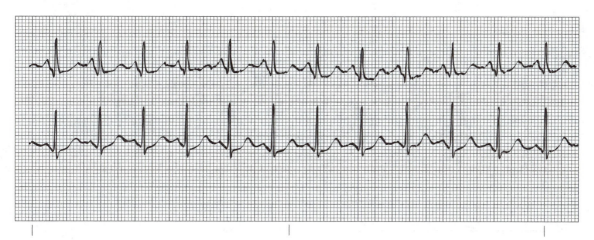

22. Rate: _____

    Rhythm: _____

    P wave: _____

    PRI: _____

    QRS: _____

    Interpretation: _____

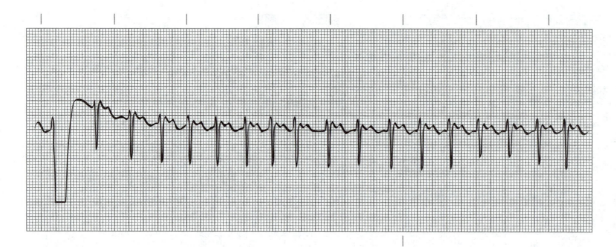

23. Rate: _____

    Rhythm: _____

    P wave: _____

    PRI: _____

    QRS: _____

    Interpretation: _____

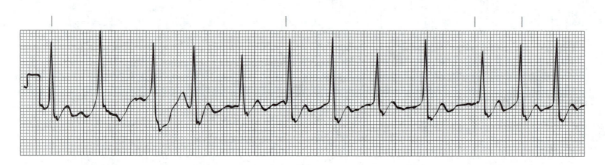

24. Rate: _____

    Rhythm: _____

    P wave: _____

    PRI: _____

    QRS: _____

    Interpretation: _____

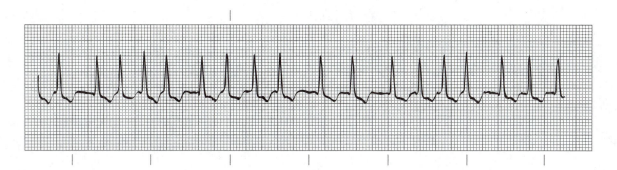

25. Rate: _____

    Rhythm: _____

    P wave: _____

    PRI: _____

    QRS: _____

    Interpretation: _____

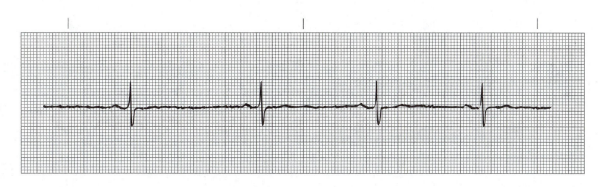

26. Rate: _____

    Rhythm: _____

    P wave: _____

    PRI: _____

    QRS: _____

    Interpretation: _____

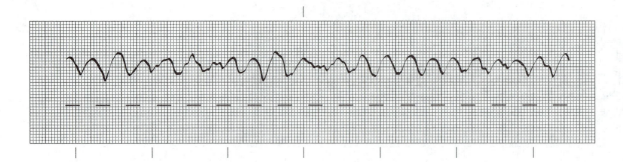

27. Rate: _____

    Rhythm: _____

    P wave: _____

    PRI: _____

    QRS: _____

    Interpretation: _____

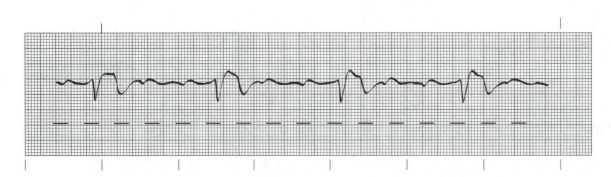

28. Rate: _____

    Rhythm: _____

    P wave: _____

    PRI: _____

    QRS: _____

    Interpretation: _____

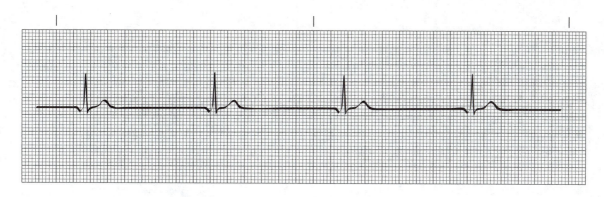

29. Rate: _____

 Rhythm: _____

 P wave: _____

 PRI: _____

 QRS: _____

 Interpretation: _____

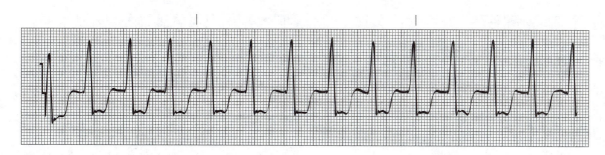

30. Rate: _____

 Rhythm: _____

 P wave: _____

 PRI: _____

 QRS: _____

 Interpretation: _____

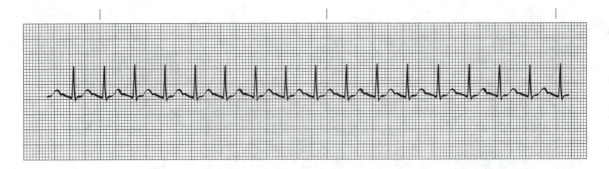

31. Rate: _____

    Rhythm: _____

    P wave: _____

    PRI: _____

    QRS: _____

    Interpretation: _____

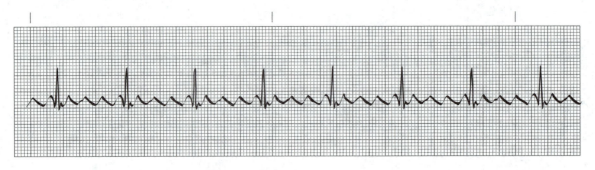

32. Rate: _____

    Rhythm: _____

    P wave: _____

    PRI: _____

    QRS: _____

    Interpretation: _____

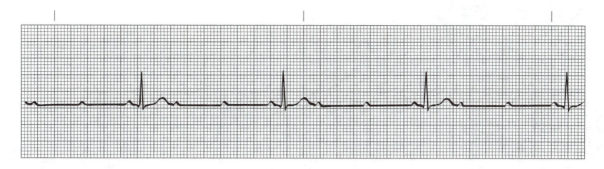

33. Rate: _____

    Rhythm: _____

    P wave: _____

    PRI: _____

    QRS: _____

    Interpretation: _____

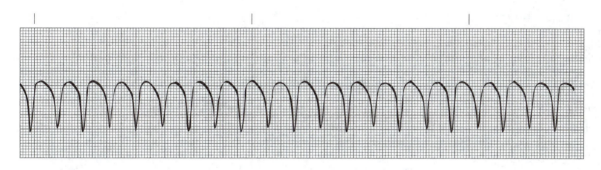

34. Rate: _____

    Rhythm: _____

    P wave: _____

    PRI: _____

    QRS: _____

    Interpretation: _____

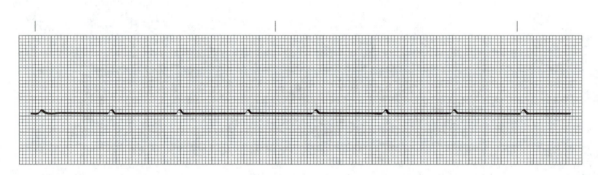

35. Rate: _____

    Rhythm: _____

    P wave: _____

    PRI: _____

    QRS: _____

    Interpretation: _____

36. Rate: _____

    Rhythm: _____

    P wave: _____

    PRI: _____

    QRS: _____

    Interpretation: _____

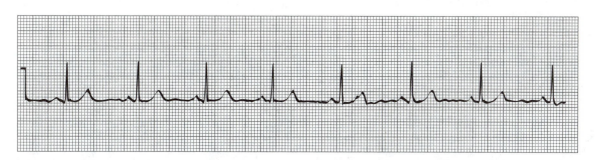

37. Rate: _____

    Rhythm: _____

    P wave: _____

    PRI: _____

    QRS: _____

    Interpretation: _____

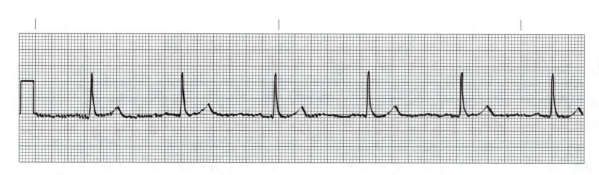

38. Rate: _____

    Rhythm: _____

    P wave: _____

    PRI: _____

    QRS: _____

    Interpretation: _____

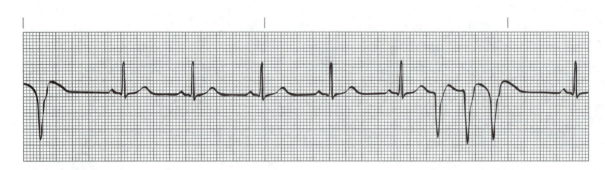

39. Rate: _____

    Rhythm: _____

    P wave: _____

    PRI: _____

    QRS: _____

    Interpretation: _____

40. Rate: _____

    Rhythm: _____

    P wave: _____

    PRI: _____

    QRS: _____

    Interpretation: _____

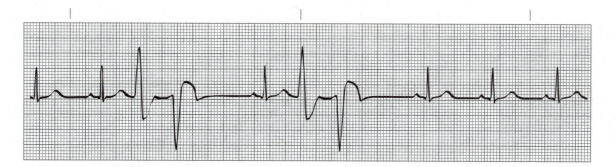

41. Rate: _____

    Rhythm: _____

    P wave: _____

    PRI: _____

    QRS: _____

    Interpretation: _____

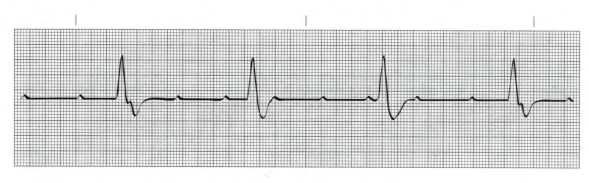

42. Rate: _____

    Rhythm: _____

    P wave: _____

    PRI: _____

    QRS: _____

    Interpretation: _____

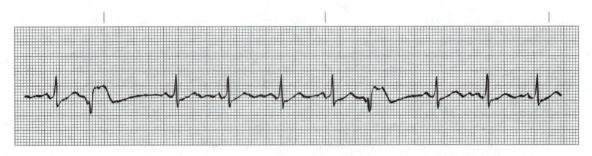

43. Rate: _____

    Rhythm: _____

    P wave: _____

    PRI: _____

    QRS: _____

    Interpretation: _____

44. Rate: _____

    Rhythm: _____

    P wave: _____

    PRI: _____

    QRS: _____

    Interpretation: _____

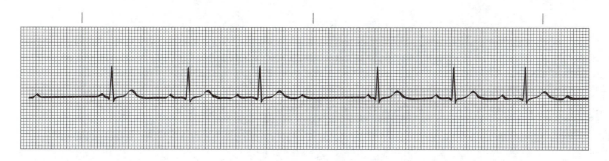

45. Rate: _____

    Rhythm: _____

    P wave: _____

    PRI: _____

    QRS: _____

    Interpretation: _____

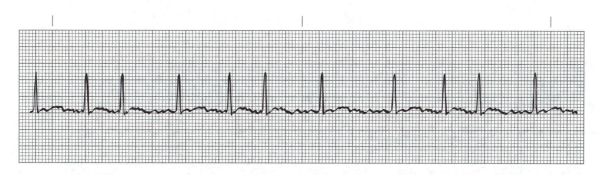

46. Rate: _____

    Rhythm: _____

    P wave: _____

    PRI: _____

    QRS: _____

    Interpretation: _____

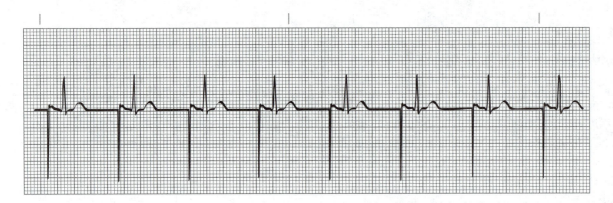

47. Rate: _____

    Rhythm: _____

    P wave: _____

    PRI: _____

    QRS: _____

    Interpretation: _____

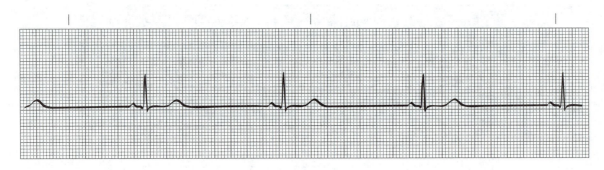

48. Rate: _____

    Rhythm: _____

    P wave: _____

    PRI: _____

    QRS: _____

    Interpretation: _____

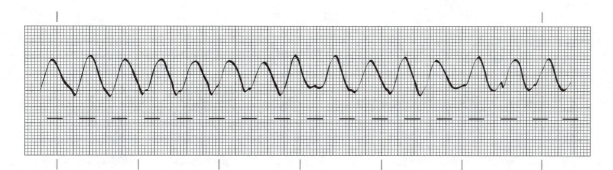

49. Rate: _____

    Rhythm: _____

    P wave: _____

    PRI: _____

    QRS: _____

    Interpretation: _____

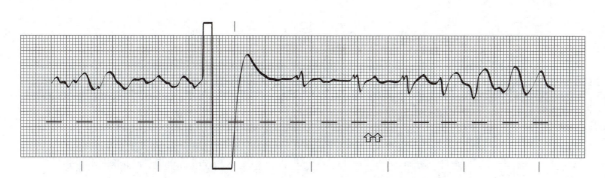

50. Rate: _____

    Rhythm: _____

    P wave: _____

    PRI: _____

    QRS: _____

    Interpretation: _____

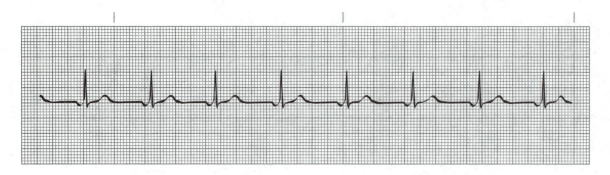

51. Rate: _____

    Rhythm: _____

    P wave: _____

    PRI: _____

    QRS: _____

    Interpretation: _____

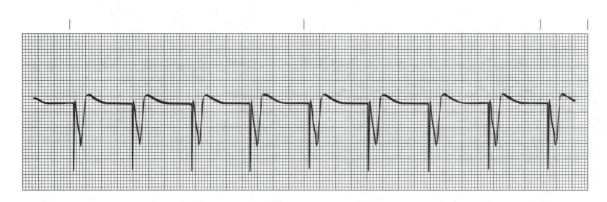

52. Rate: _____

    Rhythm: _____

    P wave: _____

    PRI: _____

    QRS: _____

    Interpretation: _____

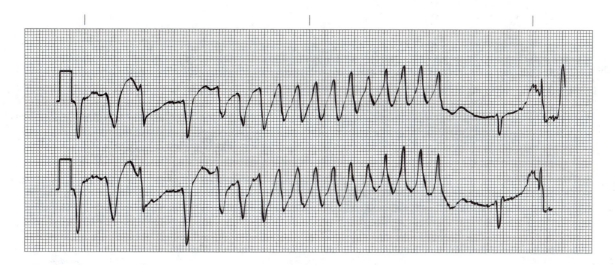

53. Rate: _____

    Rhythm: _____

    P waves:_____

    PRI: _____

    QRS: _____

    Interpretation: _____

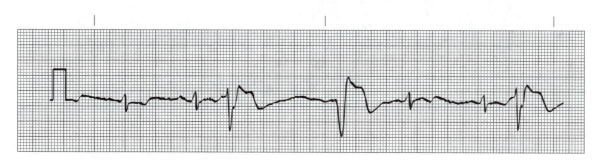

54. Rate: _____

    Rhythm: _____

    P wave: _____

    PRI: _____

    QRS: _____

    Interpretation: _____

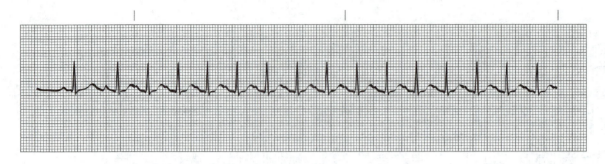

55. Rate: _____

    Rhythm: _____

    P wave: _____

    PRI: _____

    QRS: _____

    Interpretation: _____

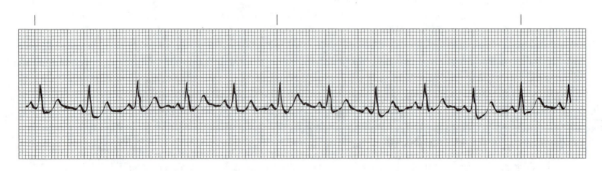

56. Rate: _____

    Rhythm: _____

    P wave: _____

    PRI: _____

    QRS: _____

    Interpretation: _____

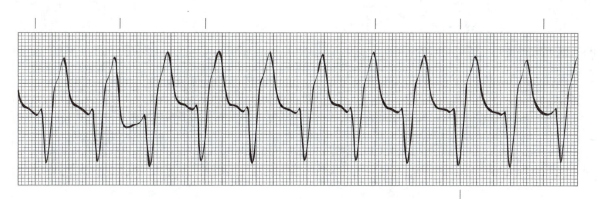

57. Rate: _____

    Rhythm: _____

    P wave: _____

    PRI: _____

    QRS: _____

    Interpretation: _____

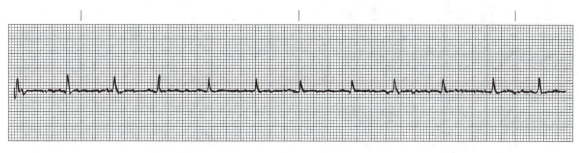

58. Rate: _____

    Rhythm: _____

    P wave: _____

    PRI: _____

    QRS: _____

    Interpretation: _____

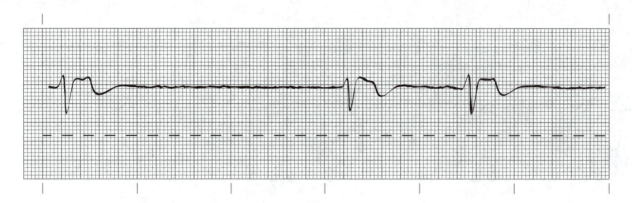

59. Rate: _____
    Rhythm: _____
    P wave: _____
    PRI: _____
    QRS: _____

    Interpretation: _____

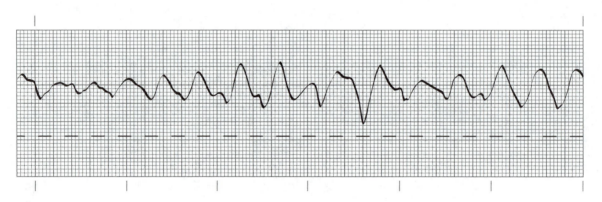

60. Rate: _____
    Rhythm: _____
    P wave: _____
    PRI: _____
    QRS: _____

    Interpretation: _____

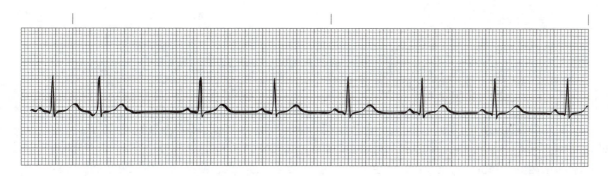

61. Rate: _____

 Rhythm: _____

 P wave: _____

 PRI: _____

 QRS: _____

 Interpretation: _____

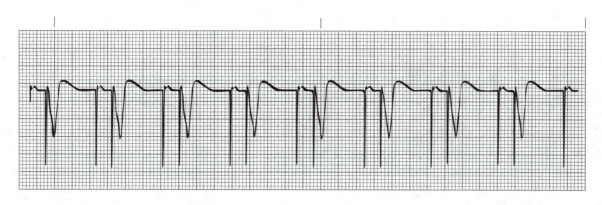

62. Rate: _____

 Rhythm: _____

 P wave: _____

 PRI: _____

 QRS: _____

 Interpretation: _____

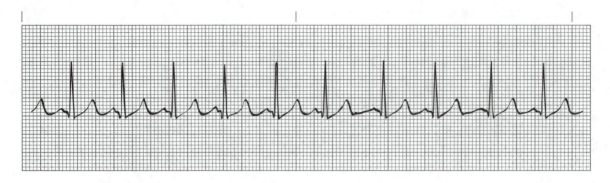

63. Rate: _____

    Rhythm: _____

    P wave: _____

    PRI: _____

    QRS: _____

    Interpretation: _____

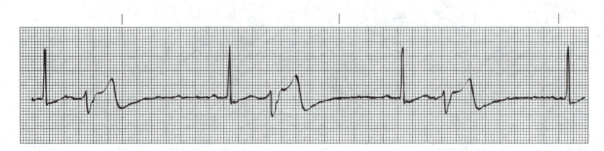

64. Rate: _____

    Rhythm: _____

    P wave: _____

    PRI: _____

    QRS: _____

    Interpretation: _____

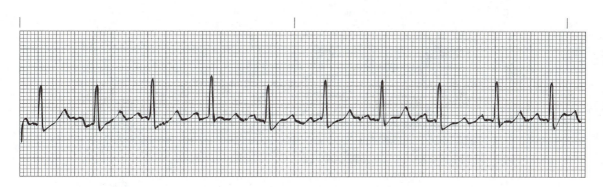

65. Rate: _____

    Rhythm: _____

    P wave: _____

    PRI: _____

    QRS: _____

    Interpretation: _____

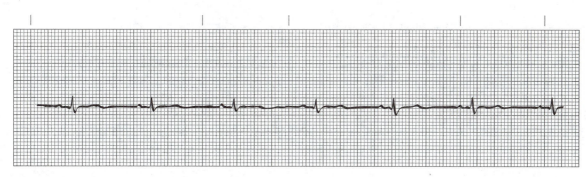

66. Rate: _____

    Rhythm: _____

    P wave: _____

    PRI: _____

    QRS: _____

    Interpretation: _____

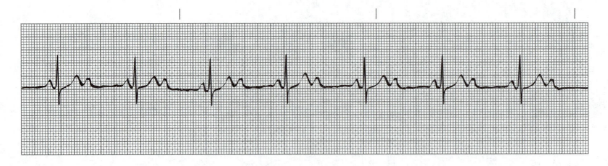

67. Rate: _____

    Rhythm: _____

    P wave: _____

    PRI: _____

    QRS: _____

    Interpretation: _____

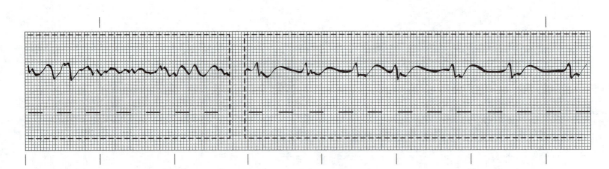

68. Rate: _____

    Rhythm: _____

    P wave: _____

    PRI: _____

    QRS: _____

    Interpretation: _____

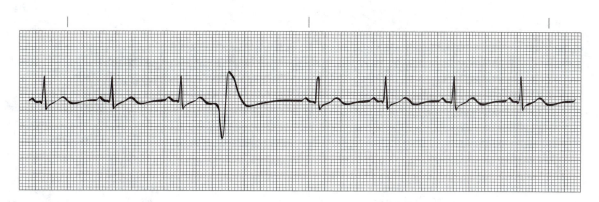

69. Rate: _____

    Rhythm: _____

    P wave: _____

    PRI: _____

    QRS: _____

    Interpretation: _____

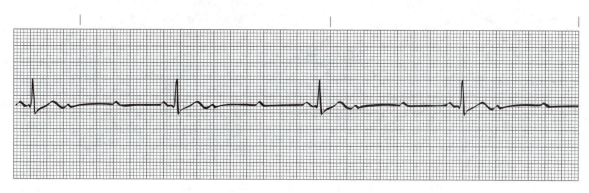

70. Rate: _____

    Rhythm: _____

    P wave: _____

    PRI: _____

    QRS: _____

    Interpretation: _____

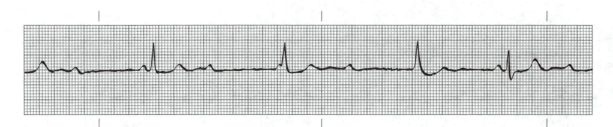

71. Rate: _____

    Rhythm: _____

    P wave: _____

    PRI: _____

    QRS: _____

    Interpretation: _____

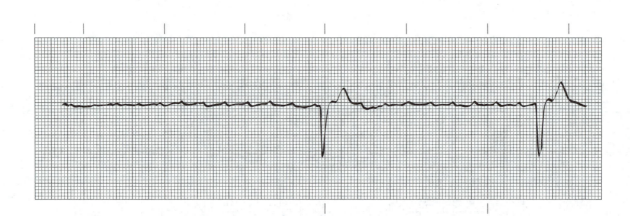

72. Rate: _____

    Rhythm: _____

    P wave: _____

    PRI: _____

    QRS: _____

    Interpretation: _____

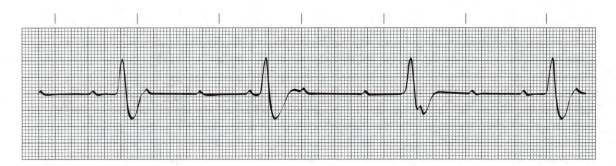

73. Rate: _____

    Rhythm: _____

    P wave: _____

    PRI: _____

    QRS: _____

    Interpretation: _____

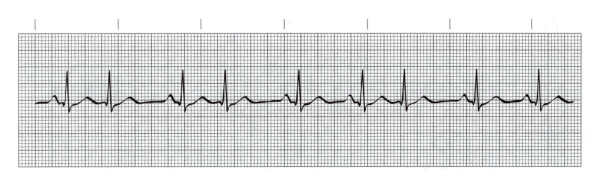

74. Rate: _____

    Rhythm: _____

    P waves:_____

    PRI: _____

    QRS: _____

    Interpretation: _____

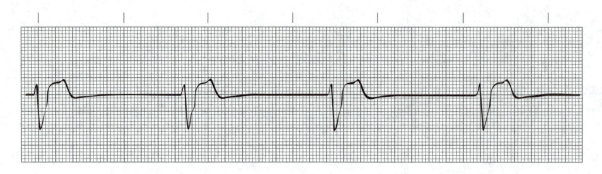

75. Rate: _____

    Rhythm: _____

    P wave: _____

    PRI: _____

    QRS: _____

    Interpretation: _____

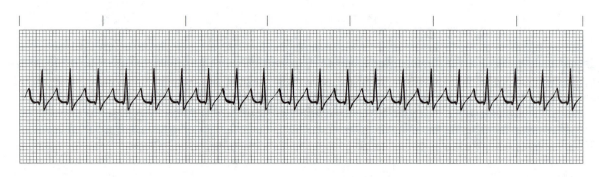

76. Rate: _____

    Rhythm: _____

    P wave: _____

    PRI: _____

    QRS: _____

    Interpretation: _____

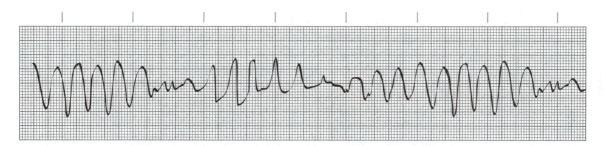

77. Rate: _____

    Rhythm: _____

    P wave: _____

    PRI: _____

    QRS: _____

    Interpretation: _____

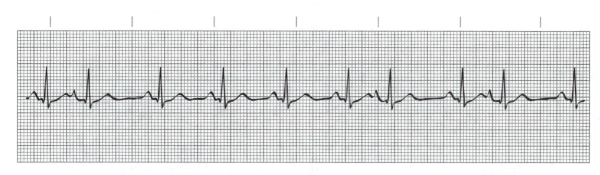

78. Rate: _____

    Rhythm: _____

    P wave: _____

    PRI: _____

    QRS: _____

    Interpretation: _____

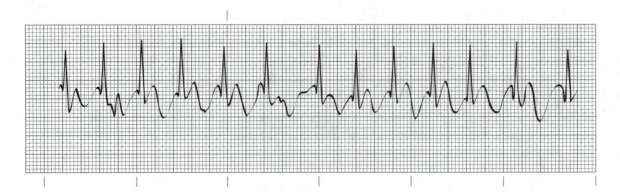

79. Rate: _____

    Rhythm: _____

    P wave: _____

    PRI: _____

    QRS: _____

    Interpretation: _____

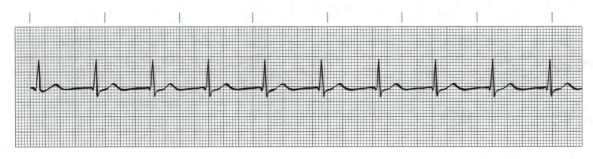

80. Rate: _____

    Rhythm: _____

    P wave: _____

    PRI: _____

    QRS: _____

    Interpretation: _____

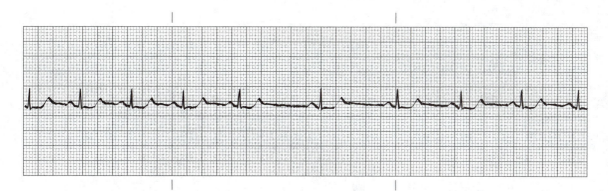

81. Rate: _____
    Rhythm: _____
    P wave: _____
    PRI: _____
    QRS: _____

    Interpretation: _____

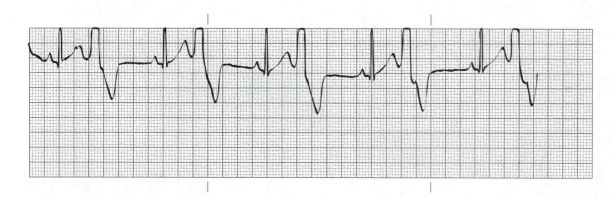

82. Rate: _____
    Rhythm: _____
    P wave: _____
    PRI: _____
    QRS: _____

    Interpretation: _____

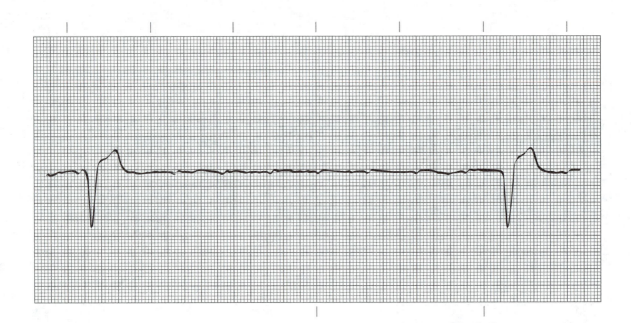

83. Rate: _____

    Rhythm: _____

    P wave: _____

    PRI: _____

    QRS: _____

    Interpretation: _____

84. Rate: _____

    Rhythm: _____

    P wave: _____

    PRI: _____

    QRS: _____

    Interpretation: _____

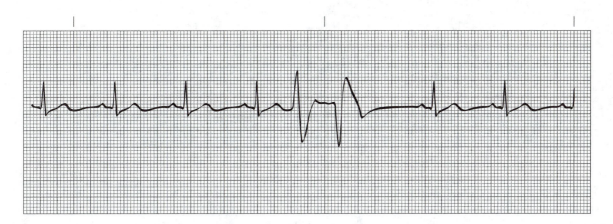

85. Rate: _____

    Rhythm: _____

    P wave: _____

    PRI: _____

    QRS: _____

    Interpretation: _____

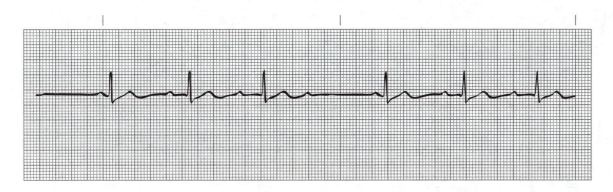

86. Rate: _____

    Rhythm: _____

    P wave: _____

    PRI: _____

    QRS: _____

    Interpretation: _____

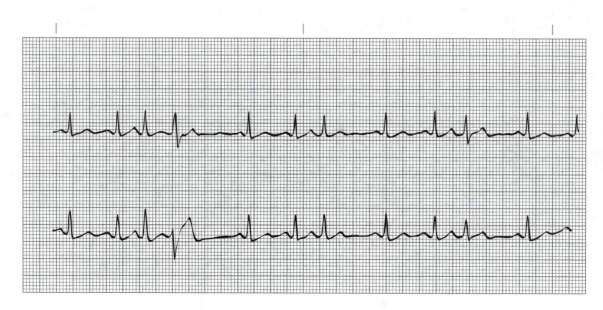

87. Rate: _____

    Rhythm: _____

    P wave: _____

    PRI: _____

    QRS: _____

    Interpretation: _____

88. Rate: _____

    Rhythm: _____

    P wave: _____

    PRI: _____

    QRS: _____

    Interpretation: _____

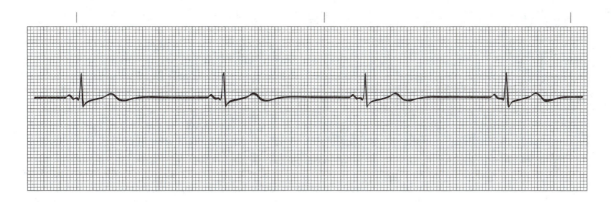

89. Rate: _____

    Rhythm: _____

    P wave: _____

    PRI: _____

    QRS: _____

    Interpretation: _____

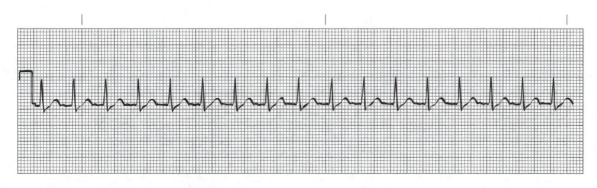

90. Rate: _____

    Rhythm: _____

    P wave: _____

    PRI: _____

    QRS: _____

    Interpretation: _____

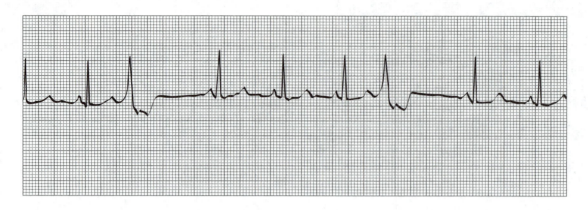

91. Rate: _____

    Rhythm: _____

    P wave: _____

    PRI: _____

    QRS: _____

    Interpretation: _____

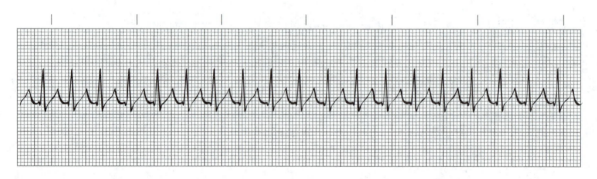

92. Rate: _____

    Rhythm: _____

    P wave: _____

    PRI: _____

    QRS: _____

    Interpretation: _____

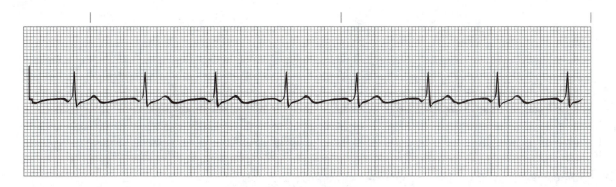

93. Rate: _____

    Rhythm: _____

    P wave: _____

    PRI: _____

    QRS: _____

    Interpretation: _____

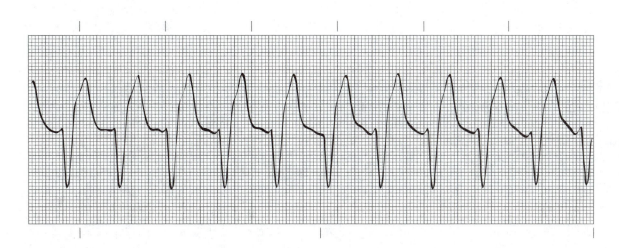

94. Rate: _____

    Rhythm: _____

    P wave: _____

    PRI: _____

    QRS: _____

    Interpretation: _____

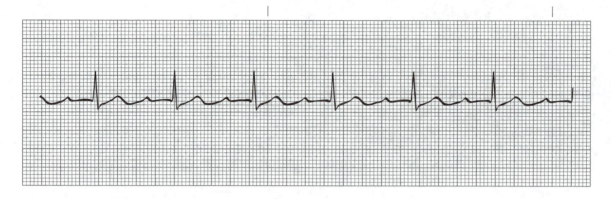

95. Rate: _____

    Rhythm: _____

    P wave: _____

    PRI: _____

    QRS: _____

    Interpretation: _____

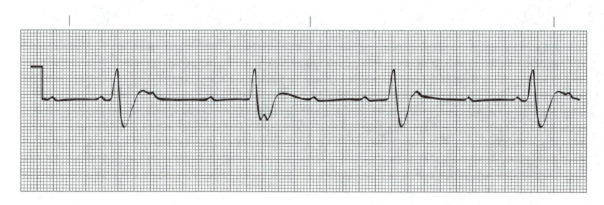

96. Rate: _____

    Rhythm: _____

    P wave: _____

    PRI: _____

    QRS: _____

    Interpretation: _____

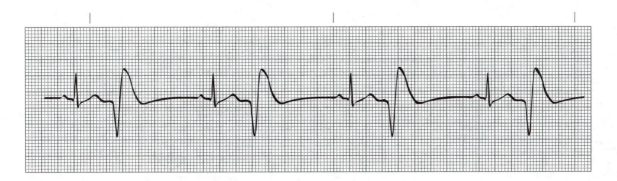

97. Rate: _____

    Rhythm: _____

    P wave: _____

    PRI: _____

    QRS: _____

    Interpretation: _____

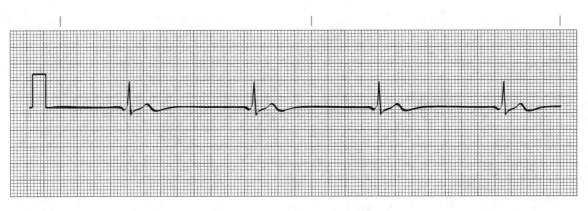

98. Rate: _____

    Rhythm: _____

    P wave: _____

    PRI: _____

    QRS: _____

    Interpretation: _____

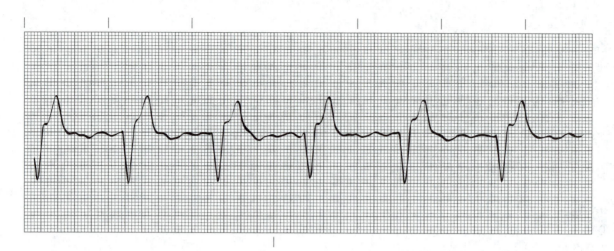

99. Rate: _____

    Rhythm: _____

    P wave: _____

    PRI: _____

    QRS: _____

    Interpretation: _____

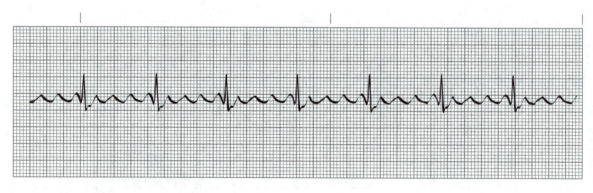

100. Rate: _____

    Rhythm: _____

    P wave: _____

    PRI: _____

    QRS: _____

    Interpretation: _____

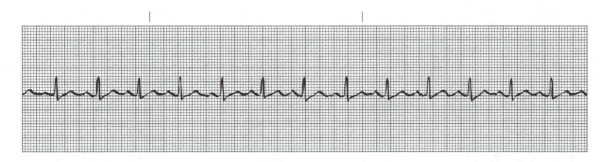

101. Rate: _____

    Rhythm: _____

    P wave: _____

    PRI: _____

    QRS: _____

    Interpretation: _____

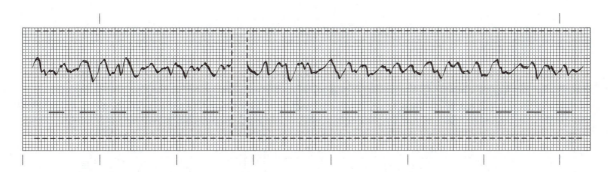

102. Rate: _____

    Rhythm: _____

    P wave: _____

    PRI: _____

    QRS: _____

    Interpretation: _____

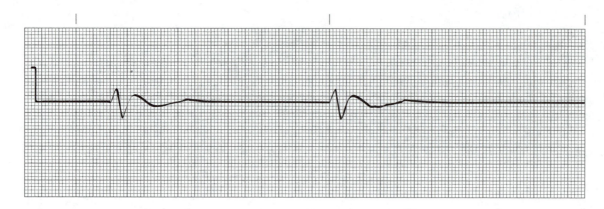

103. Rate: _____

    Rhythm: _____

    P Wave: _____

    PRI: _____

    QRS: _____

    Interpretation: _____

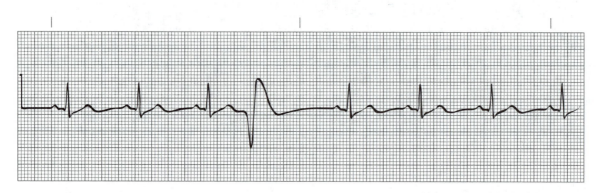

104. Rate: _____

    Rhythm: _____

    P wave: _____

    PRI: _____

    QRS: _____

    Interpretation: _____

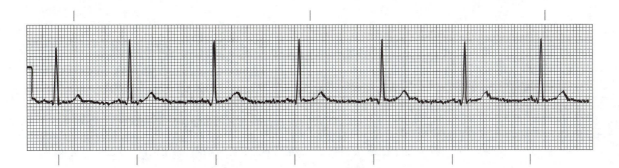

105. Rate: _____

Rhythm: _____

P wave: _____

PRI: _____

QRS: _____

Interpretation: _____

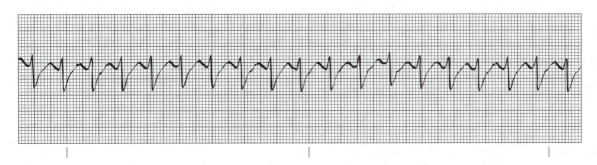

106. Rate: _____

Rhythm: _____

P wave: _____

PRI: _____

QRS: _____

Interpretation: _____

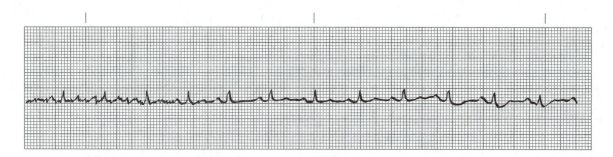

107. Rate: _____

    Rhythm: _____

    P wave: _____

    PRI: _____

    QRS: _____

    Interpretation: _____

108. Rate: _____

    Rhythm: _____

    P wave: _____

    PRI: _____

    QRS: _____

    Interpretation: _____

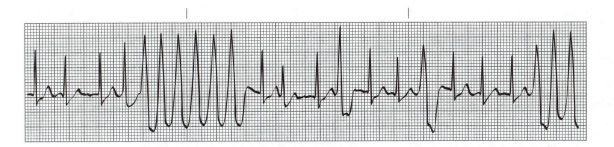

109. Rate: _____

    Rhythm: _____

    P wave: _____

    PRI: _____

    QRS: _____

    Interpretation: _____

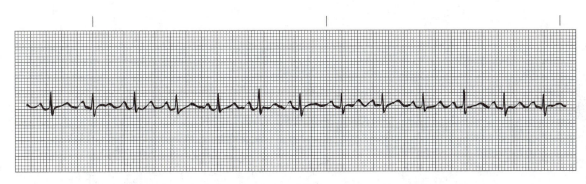

110. Rate: _____

    Rhythm: _____

    P wave: _____

    PRI: _____

    QRS: _____

    Interpretation: _____

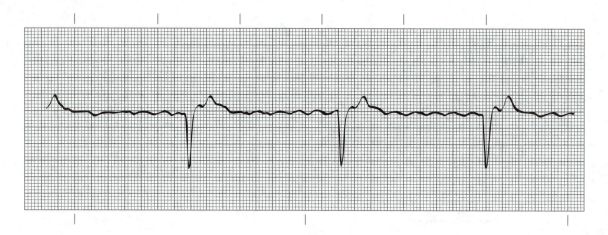

111. Rate: _____

    Rhythm: _____

    P wave: _____

    PRI: _____

    QRS: _____

    Interpretation: _____

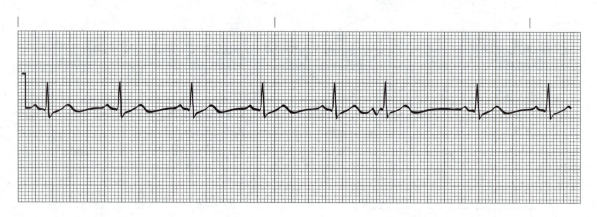

112. Rate: _____

    Rhythm: _____

    P wave: _____

    PRI: _____

    QRS: _____

    Interpretation: _____

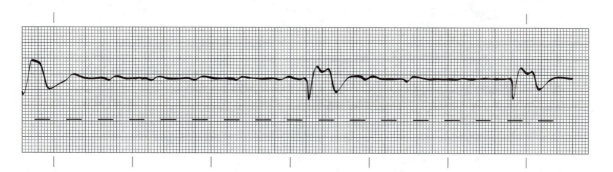

113. Rate: _____

Rhythm: _____

P wave: _____

PRI: _____

QRS: _____

Interpretation: _____

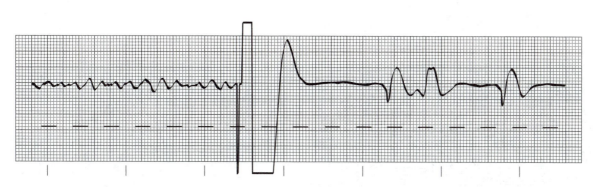

114. Rate: _____

Rhythm: _____

P wave: _____

PRI: _____

QRS: _____

Interpretation: _____

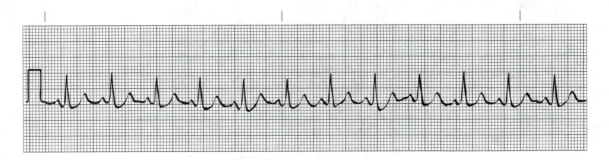

115. Rate: _____

    Rhythm: _____

    P wave: _____

    PRI: _____

    QRS: _____

    Interpretation: _____

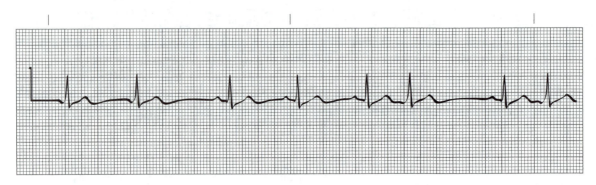

116. Rate: _____

    Rhythm: _____

    P wave: _____

    PRI: _____

    QRS: _____

    Interpretation: _____

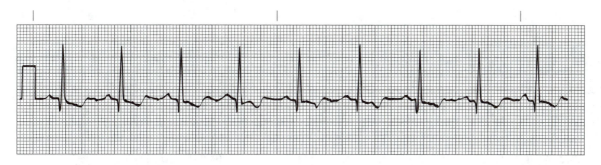

117. Rate: _____
     Rhythm: _____
     P wave: _____
     PRI: _____
     QRS: _____

     Interpretation: _____

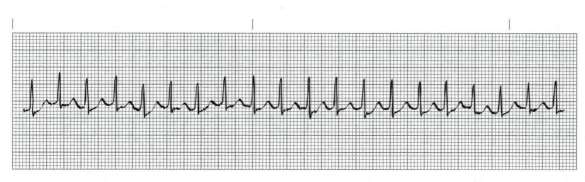

118. Rate: _____
     Rhythm: _____
     P wave: _____
     PRI: _____
     QRS: _____

     Interpretation: _____

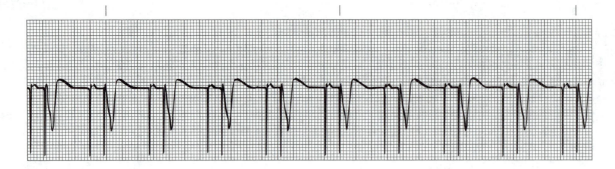

119. Rate: _____

    Rhythm: _____

    P wave: _____

    PRI: _____

    QRS: _____

    Interpretation: _____

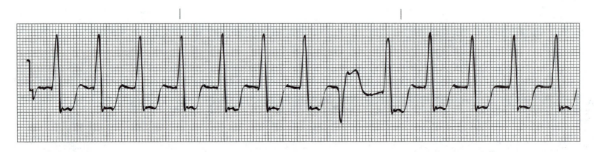

120. Rate: _____

    Rhythm: _____

    P wave: _____

    PRI: _____

    QRS: _____

    Interpretation: _____

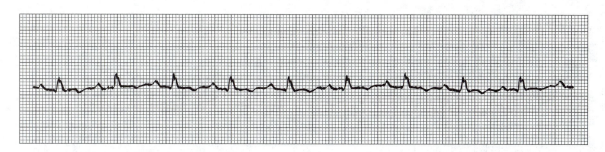

121. Rate: _____

    Rhythm: _____

    P wave: _____

    PRI: _____

    QRS: _____

    Interpretation: _____

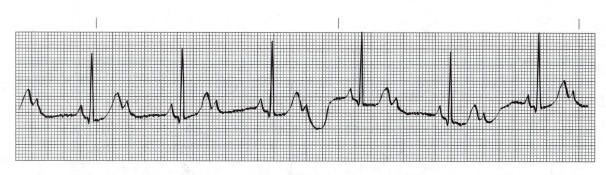

122. Rate: _____

    Rhythm: _____

    P wave: _____

    PRI: _____

    QRS: _____

    Interpretation: _____

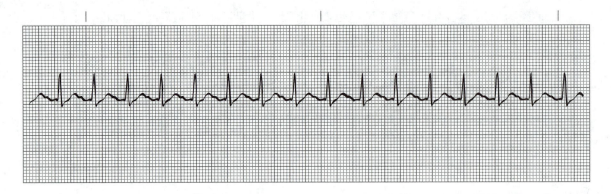

123. Rate: _____

Rhythm: _____

P wave: _____

PRI: _____

QRS: _____

Interpretation: _____

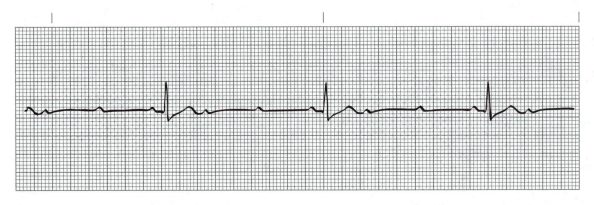

124. Rate: _____

Rhythm: _____

P wave: _____

PRI: _____

QRS: _____

Interpretation: _____

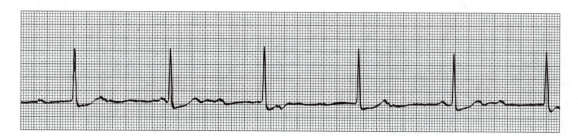

125. Rate: _____

Rhythm: _____

P wave: _____

PRI: _____

QRS: _____

Interpretation: _____

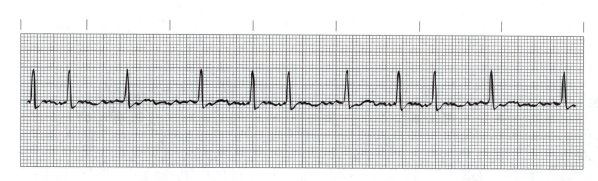

126. Rate: _____

Rhythm: _____

P wave: _____

PRI: _____

QRS: _____

Interpretation: _____

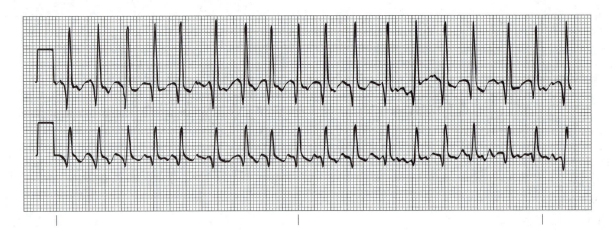

127. Rate: _____

Rhythm: _____

P wave: _____

PRI: _____

QRS: _____

Interpretation: _____

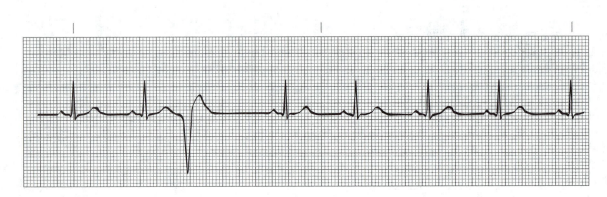

128. Rate: _____

Rhythm: _____

P wave: _____

PRI: _____

QRS: _____

Interpretation: _____

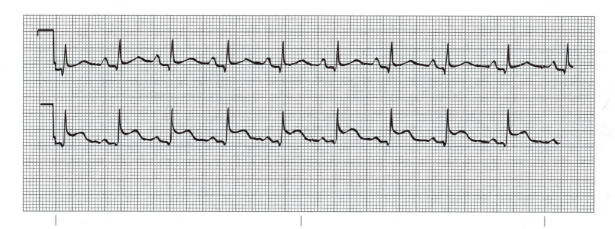

129. Rate: _____

     Rhythm: _____

     P wave: _____

     PRI: _____

     QRS: _____

     Interpretation: _____

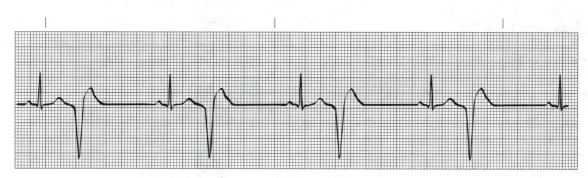

130. Rate: _____

     Rhythm: _____

     P wave: _____

     PRI: _____

     QRS: _____

     Interpretation: _____

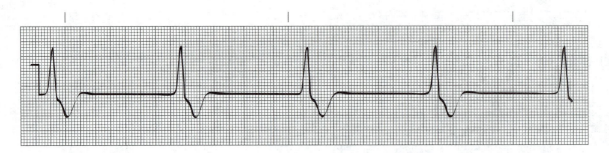

131. Rate: _____

     Rhythm: _____

     P wave: _____

     PRI: _____

     QRS: _____

     Interpretation: _____

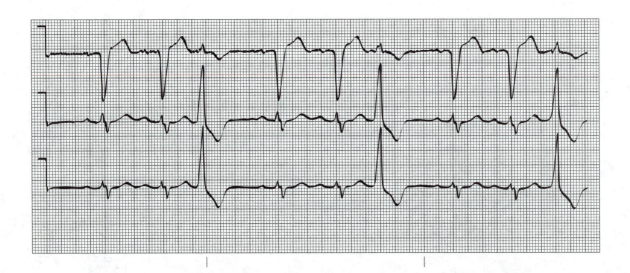

132. Rate: _____

     Rhythm: _____

     P wave: _____

     PRI: _____

     QRS: _____

     Interpretation: _____

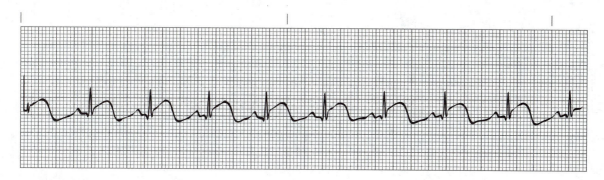

133. Rate: _____

    Rhythm: _____

    P wave: _____

    PRI: _____

    QRS: _____

    Interpretation: _____

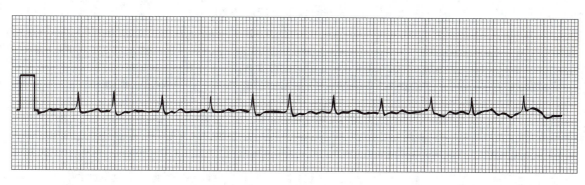

134. Rate: _____

    Rhythm: _____

    P wave: _____

    PRI: _____

    QRS: _____

    Interpretation: _____

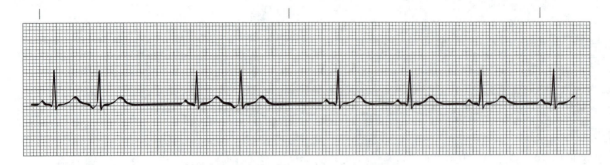

135. Rate: _____

    Rhythm: _____

    P wave: _____

    PRI: _____

    QRS: _____

    Interpretation: _____

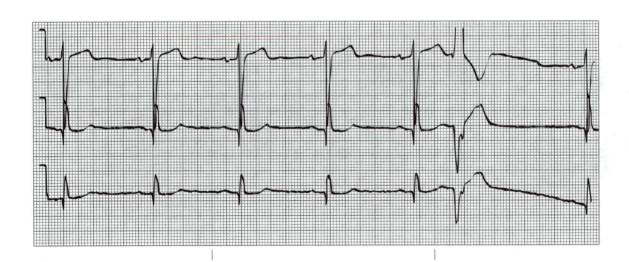

136. Rate: _____

    Rhythm: _____

    P wave: _____

    PRI: _____

    QRS: _____

    Interpretation: _____

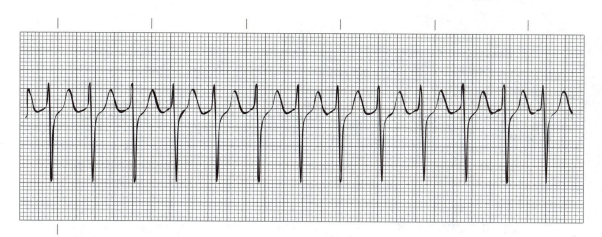

137. Rate: _____

     Rhythm: _____

     P wave: _____

     PRI: _____

     QRS: _____

     Interpretation: _____

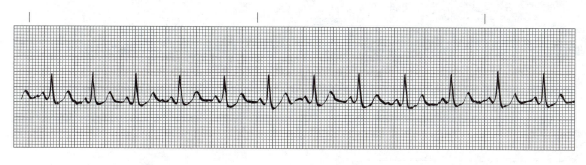

138. Rate: _____

     Rhythm: _____

     P wave: _____

     PRI: _____

     QRS: _____

     Interpretation: _____

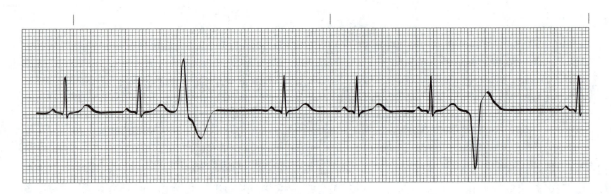

139. Rate: _____

    Rhythm: _____

    P wave: _____

    PRI: _____

    QRS: _____

    Interpretation: _____

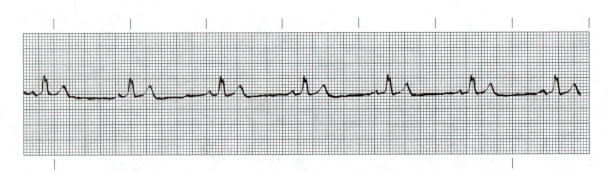

140. Rate: _____

    Rhythm: _____

    P wave: _____

    PRI: _____

    QRS: _____

    Interpretation: _____

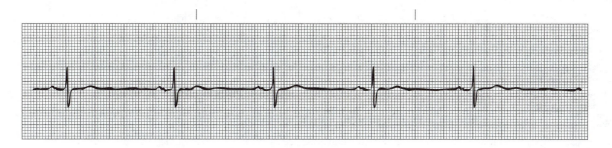

141. Rate: _____
     Rhythm: _____
     P wave: _____
     PRI: _____
     QRS: _____

     Interpretation: _____

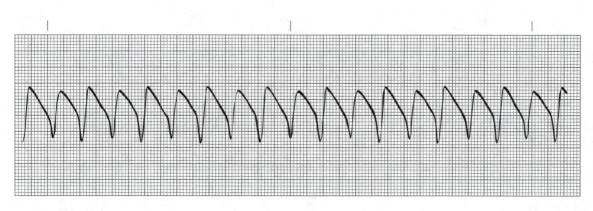

142. Rate: _____
     Rhythm: _____
     P wave: _____
     PRI: _____
     QRS: _____

     Interpretation: _____

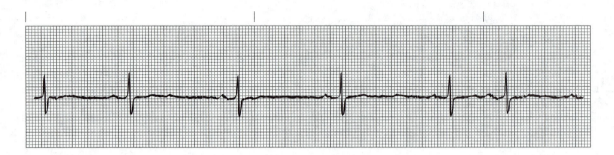

143. Rate: _____

    Rhythm: _____

    P wave: _____

    PRI: _____

    QRS: _____

    Interpretation: _____

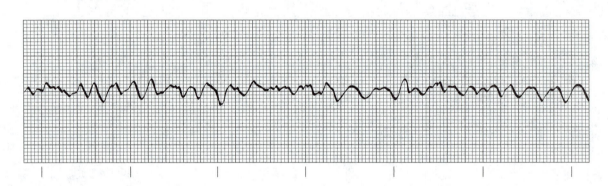

144. Rate: _____

    Rhythm: _____

    P wave: _____

    PRI: _____

    QRS: _____

    Interpretation: _____

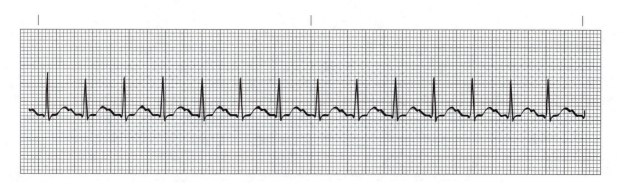

145. Rate: _____

Rhythm: _____

P wave: _____

PRI: _____

QRS: _____

Interpretation: _____

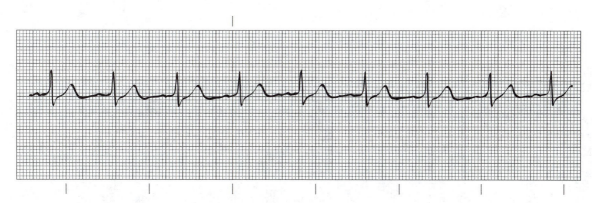

146. Rate: _____

Rhythm: _____

P wave: _____

PRI: _____

QRS: _____

Interpretation: _____

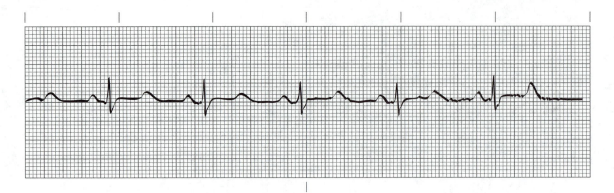

147. Rate: _____

    Rhythm: _____

    P wave: _____

    PRI: _____

    QRS: _____

    Interpretation: _____

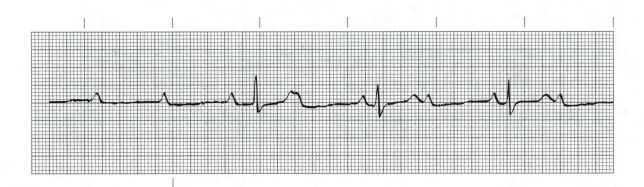

148. Rate: _____

    Rhythm: _____

    P wave: _____

    PRI: _____

    QRS: _____

    Interpretation: _____

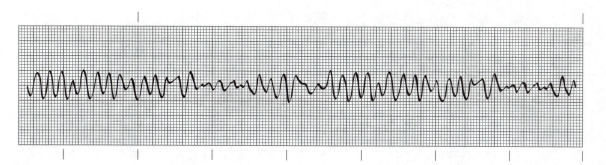

149. Rate: _____

     Rhythm: _____

     P wave: _____

     PRI: _____

     QRS: _____

     Interpretation: _____

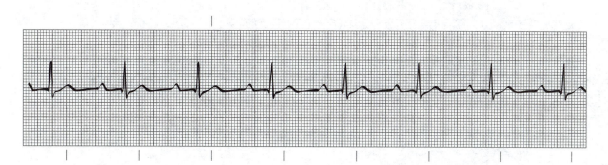

150. Rate: _____

     Rhythm: _____

     P wave: _____

     PRI: _____

     QRS: _____

     Interpretation: _____

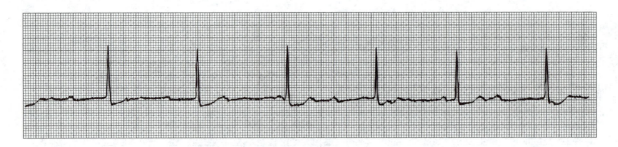

151. Rate: _____

     Rhythm: _____

     P wave: _____

     PRI: _____

     QRS: _____

     Interpretation: _____

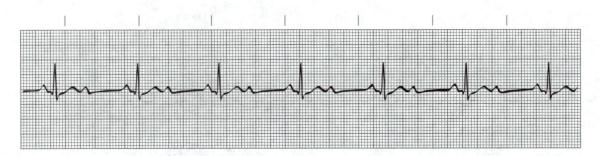

152. Rate: _____

     Rhythm: _____

     P wave: _____

     PRI: _____

     QRS: _____

     Interpretation: _____

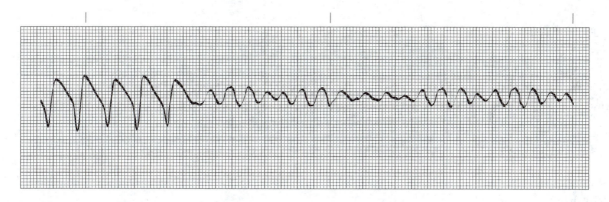

153. Rate: _____

    Rhythm: _____

    P wave: _____

    PRI: _____

    QRS: _____

    Interpretation: _____

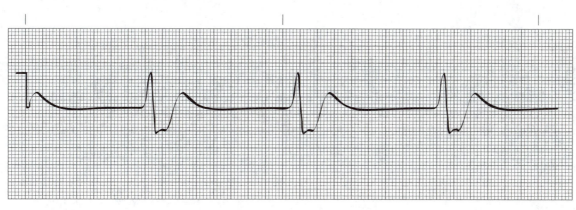

154. Rate: _____

    Rhythm: _____

    P wave: _____

    PRI: _____

    QRS: _____

    Interpretation: _____

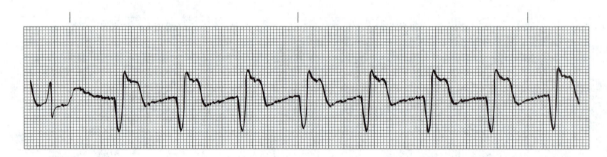

155. Rate: _____

    Rhythm: _____

    P wave: _____

    PRI: _____

    QRS: _____

    Interpretation: _____

156. Rate: _____

    Rhythm: _____

    P wave: _____

    PRI: _____

    QRS: _____

    Interpretation: _____

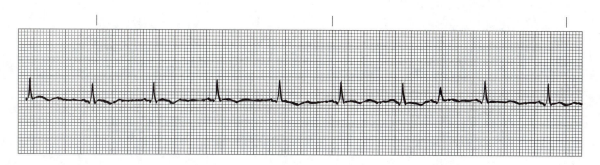

157. Rate: _____

Rhythm: _____

P wave: _____

PRI: _____

QRS: _____

Interpretation: _____

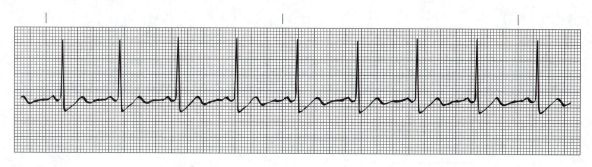

158. Rate: _____

Rhythm: _____

P wave: _____

PRI: _____

QRS: _____

Interpretation: _____

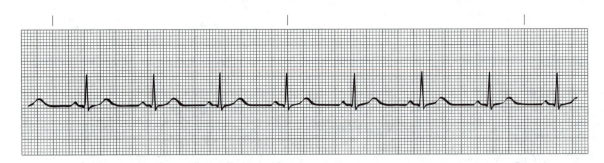

159. Rate: _____

    Rhythm: _____

    P wave: _____

    PRI: _____

    QRS: _____

    Interpretation: _____

160. Rate: _____

    Rhythm: _____

    P wave: _____

    PRI: _____

    QRS: _____

    Interpretation: _____

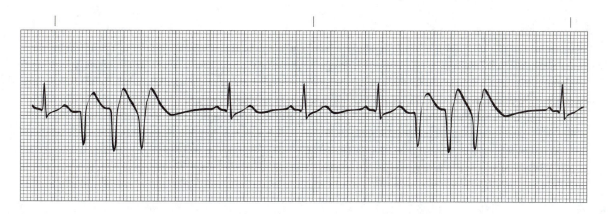

161. Rate: _____
    Rhythm: _____
    P Wave: _____
    PRI: _____
    QRS: _____

    Interpretation: _____

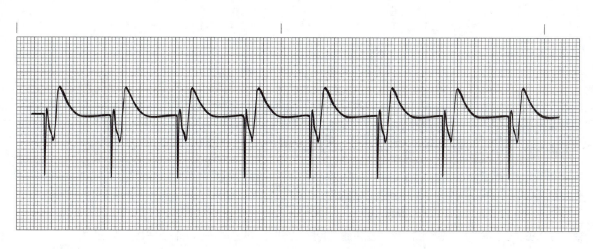

162. Rate: _____
    Rhythm: _____
    P wave: _____
    PRI: _____
    QRS: _____

    Interpretation: _____

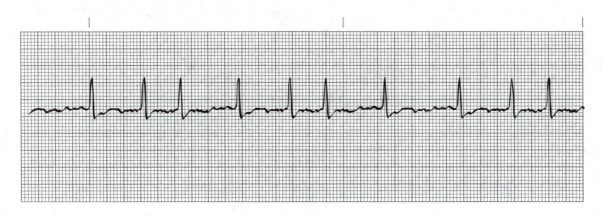

163. Rate: _____

    Rhythm: _____

    P wave: _____

    PRI: _____

    QRS: _____

    Interpretation: _____

164. Rate: _____

    Rhythm: _____

    P wave: _____

    PRI: _____

    QRS: _____

    Interpretation: _____

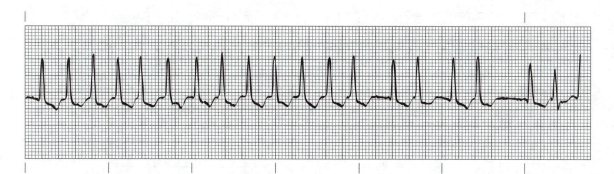

165. Rate: _____

     Rhythm: _____

     P wave: _____

     PRI: _____

     QRS: _____

     Interpretation: _____

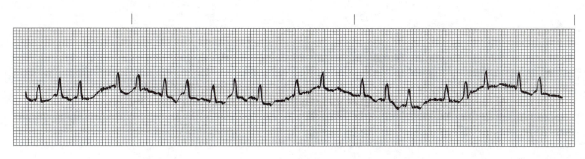

166. Rate: _____

     Rhythm: _____

     P wave: _____

     PRI: _____

     QRS: _____

     Interpretation: _____

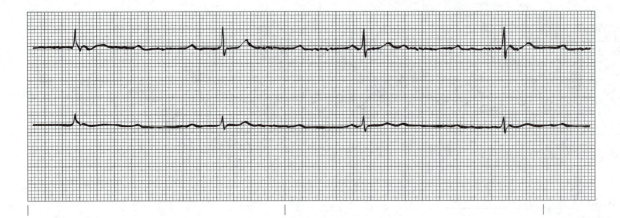

167. Rate: _____

Rhythm: _____

P wave: _____

PRI: _____

QRS: _____

Interpretation: _____

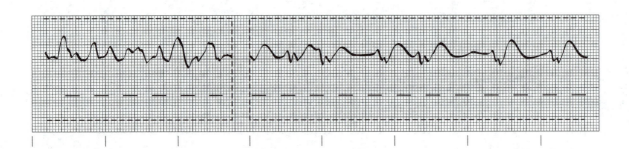

168. Rate: _____

Rhythm: _____

P wave: _____

PRI: _____

QRS: _____

Interpretation: _____

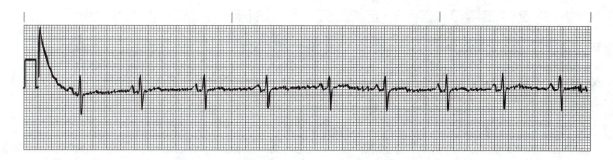

169. Rate: _____

     Rhythm: _____

     P wave: _____

     PRI: _____

     QRS: _____

     Interpretation: _____

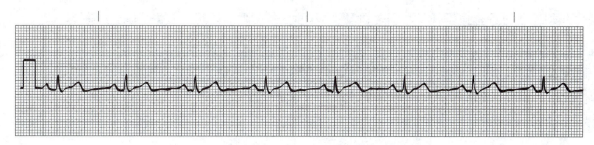

170. Rate: _____

     Rhythm: _____

     P wave: _____

     PRI: _____

     QRS: _____

     Interpretation: _____

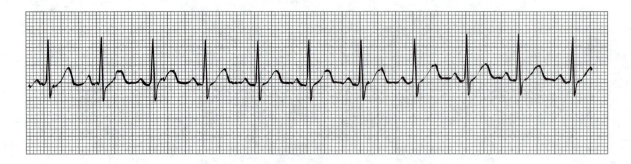

171. Rate: _____

    Rhythm: _____

    P wave: _____

    PRI: _____

    QRS: _____

    Interpretation: _____

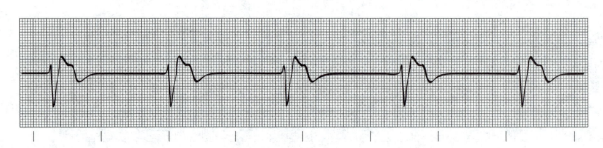

172. Rate: _____

    Rhythm: _____

    P wave: _____

    PRI: _____

    QRS: _____

    Interpretation: _____

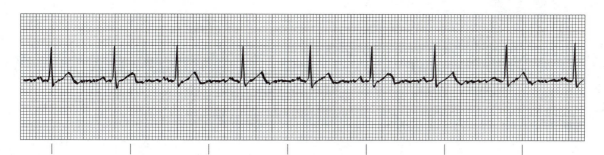

173. Rate: _____

Rhythm: _____

P Waves: _____

PRI: _____

QRS: _____

Interpretation: _____

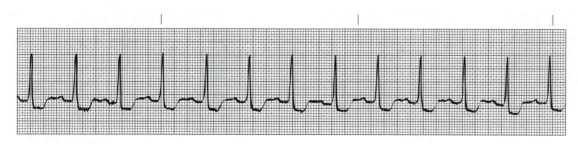

174. Rate: _____

Rhythm: _____

P wave: _____

PRI: _____

QRS: _____

Interpretation: _____

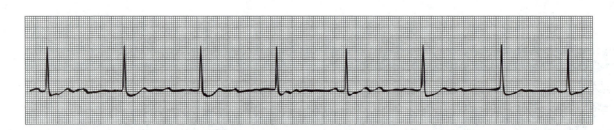

175. Rate: _____

    Rhythm: _____

    P wave: _____

    PRI: _____

    QRS: _____

    Interpretation: _____

176. Rate: _____

    Rhythm: _____

    P wave: _____

    PRI: _____

    QRS: _____

    Interpretation: _____

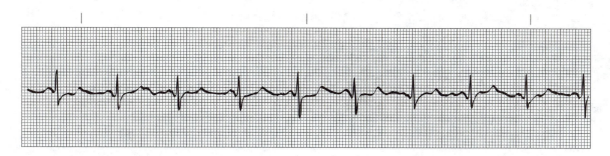

177. Rate: _____

   Rhythm: _____

   P wave: _____

   PRI: _____

   QRS: _____

   Interpretation: _____

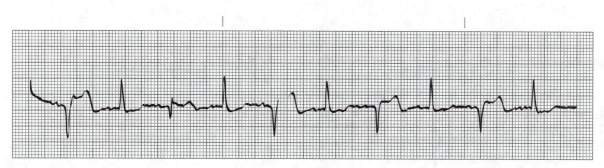

178. Rate: _____

   Rhythm: _____

   P wave: _____

   PRI: _____

   QRS: _____

   Interpretation: _____

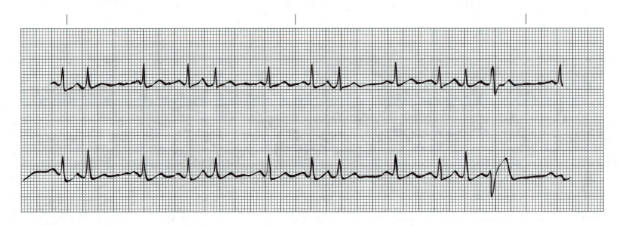

179. Rate: _____

Rhythm: _____

P wave: _____

PRI: _____

QRS: _____

Interpretation: _____

180. Rate: _____

Rhythm: _____

P wave: _____

PRI: _____

QRS: _____

Interpretation: _____

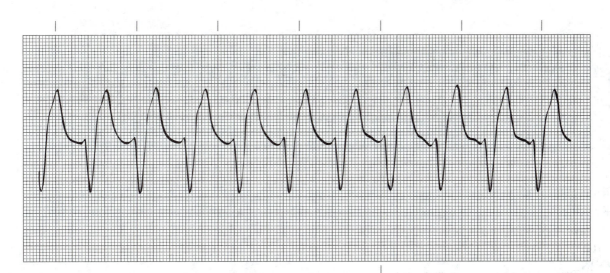

181. Rate: _____

    Rhythm: _____

    P wave: _____

    PRI: _____

    QRS: _____

    Interpretation: _____

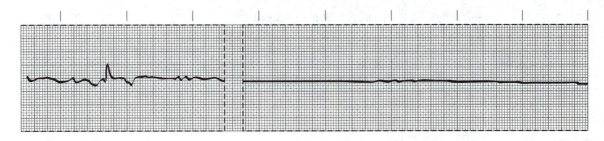

182. Rate: _____

    Rhythm: _____

    P Wave: _____

    PRI: _____

    QRS: _____

    Interpretation: _____

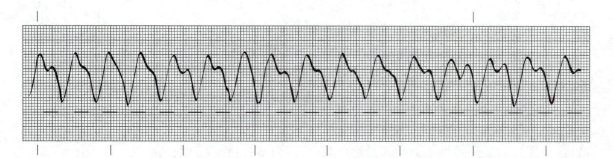

183. Rate: _____

     Rhythm: _____

     P wave: _____

     PRI: _____

     QRS: _____

     Interpretation: _____

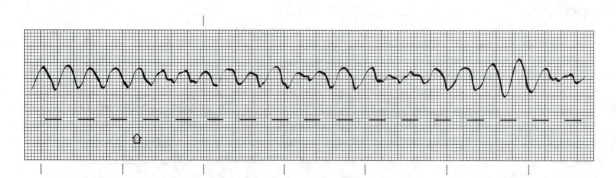

184. Rate: _____

     Rhythm: _____

     P wave: _____

     PRI: _____

     QRS: _____

     Interpretation: _____

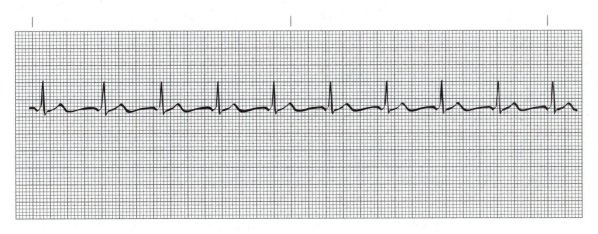

185. Rate: _____

    Rhythm: _____

    P wave: _____

    PRI: _____

    QRS: _____

    Interpretation: _____

186. Rate: _____

    Rhythm: _____

    P wave: _____

    PRI: _____

    QRS: _____

    Interpretation: _____

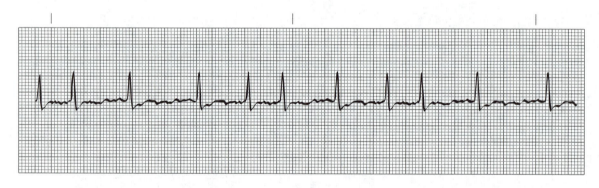

187. Rate: _____

    Rhythm: _____

    P wave: _____

    PRI: _____

    QRS: _____

    Interpretation: _____

188. Rate: _____

    Rhythm: _____

    P wave: _____

    PRI: _____

    QRS: _____

    Interpretation: _____

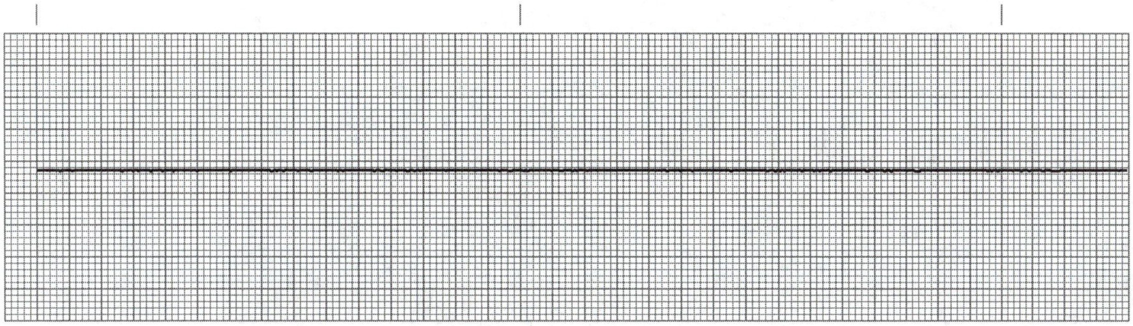

189. Rate: _____

  Rhythm: _____

  P wave: _____

  PRI: _____

  QRS: _____

  Interpretation: _____

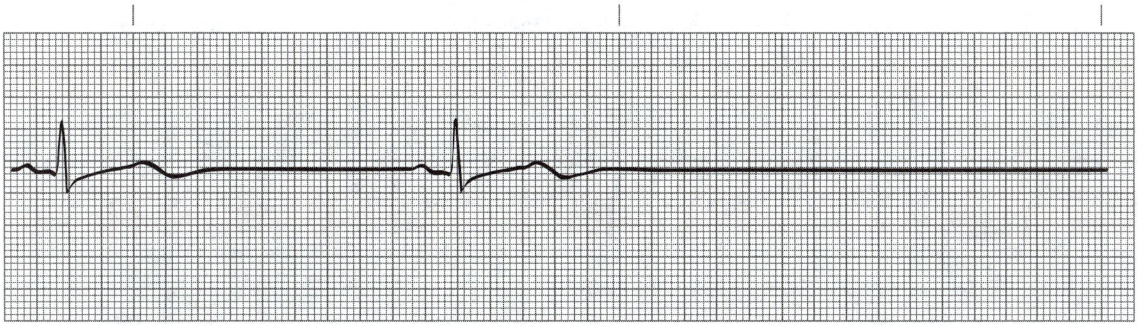

190. Rate: _____

  Rhythm: _____

  P wave: _____

  PRI: _____

  QRS: _____

  Interpretation: _____

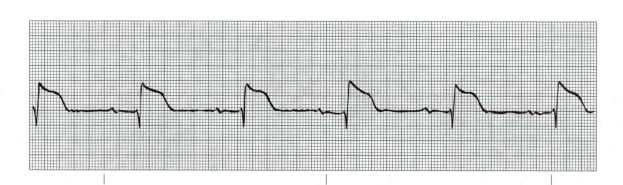

191. Rate: _____

   Rhythm: _____

   P wave: _____

   PRI: _____

   QRS: _____

   Interpretation: _____

192. Rate: _____

   Rhythm: _____

   P wave: _____

   PRI: _____

   QRS: _____

   Interpretation: _____

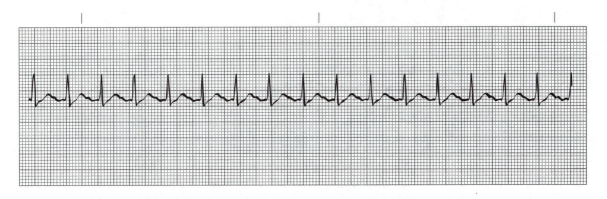

193. Rate: _____

    Rhythm: _____

    P wave: _____

    PRI: _____

    QRS: _____

    Interpretation: _____

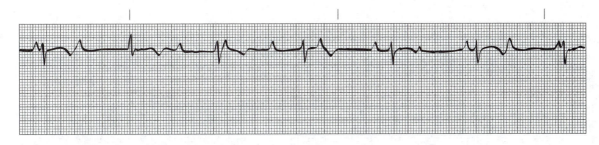

194. Rate: _____

    Rhythm: _____

    P wave: _____

    PRI: _____

    QRS: _____

    Interpretation: _____

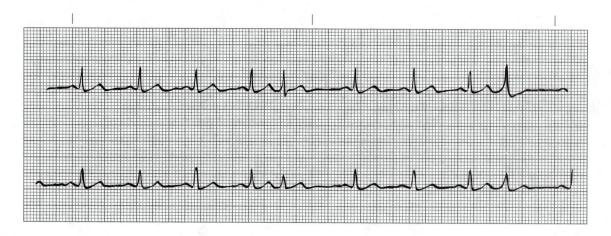

195. Rate: _____

    Rhythm: _____

    P wave: _____

    PRI: _____

    QRS: _____

    Interpretation: _____

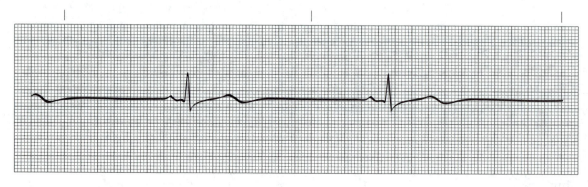

196. Rate: _____

    Rhythm: _____

    P wave: _____

    PRI: _____

    QRS: _____

    Interpretation: _____

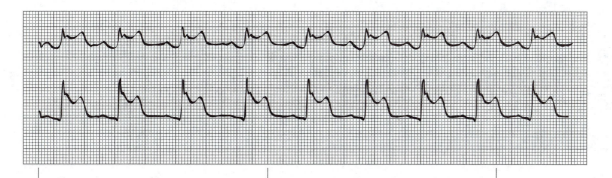

197. Rate: _____

     Rhythm: _____

     P wave: _____

     PRI: _____

     QRS: _____

     Interpretation: _____

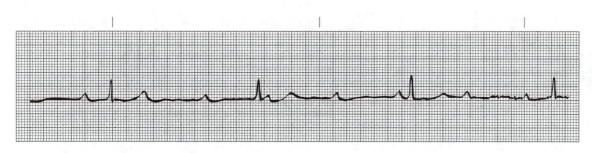

198. Rate: _____

     Rhythm: _____

     P wave: _____

     PRI: _____

     QRS: _____

     Interpretation: _____

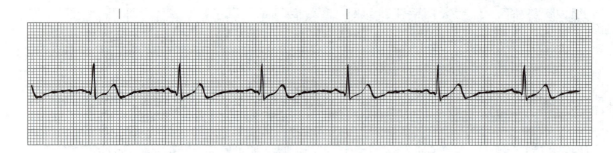

199. Rate: _____

     Rhythm: _____

     P wave: _____

     PRI: _____

     QRS: _____

     Interpretation: _____

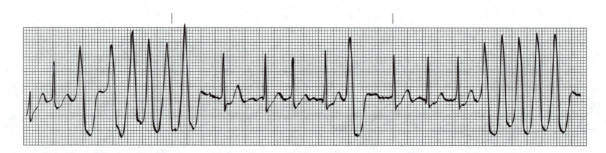

200. Rate: _____

     Rhythm: _____

     P wave: _____

     PRI: _____

     QRS: _____

     Interpretation: _____

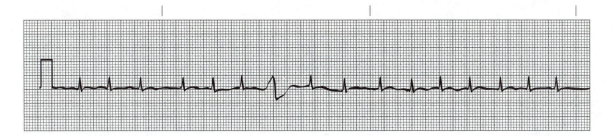

201. Rate: _____

     Rhythm: _____

     P wave: _____

     PRI: _____

     QRS: _____

     Interpretation: _____

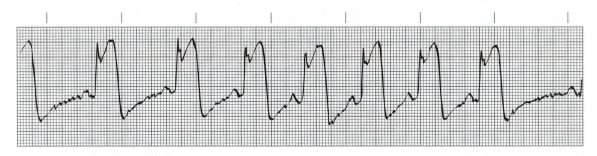

202. Rate: _____

     Rhythm: _____

     P wave: _____

     PRI: _____

     QRS: _____

     Interpretation: _____

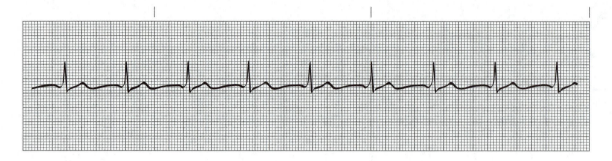

203. Rate: _____

Rhythm: _____

P wave: _____

PRI: _____

QRS: _____

Interpretation: _____

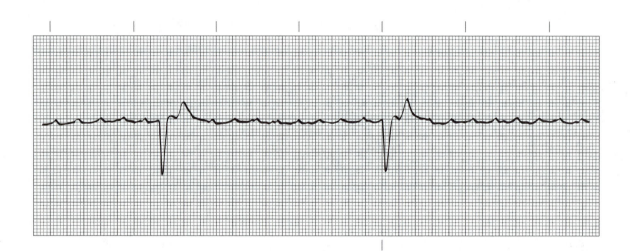

204. Rate: _____

Rhythm: _____

P wave: _____

PRI: _____

QRS: _____

Interpretation: _____

205. Rate: _____

    Rhythm: _____

    P wave: _____

    PRI: _____

    QRS: _____

    Interpretation: _____

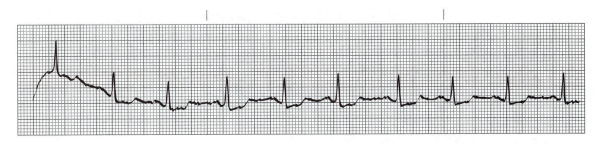

206. Rate: _____

    Rhythm: _____

    P wave: _____

    PRI: _____

    QRS: _____

    Interpretation: _____

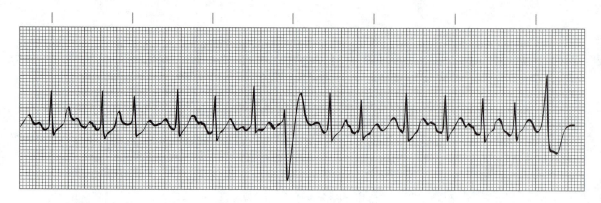

207. Rate: _____

    Rhythm: _____

    P Wave: _____

    PRI: _____

    QRS: _____

    Interpretation: _____

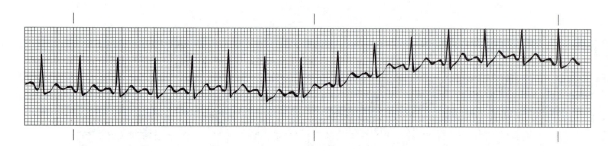

208. Rate: _____

    Rhythm: _____

    P wave: _____

    PRI: _____

    QRS: _____

    Interpretation: _____

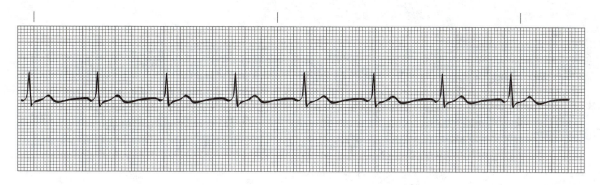

209. Rate: _____

Rhythm: _____

P wave: _____

PRI: _____

QRS: _____

Interpretation: _____

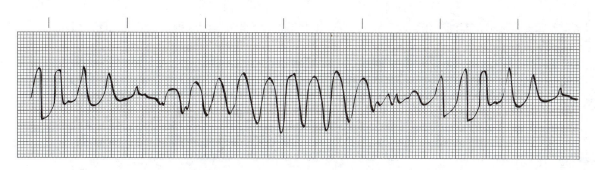

210. Rate: _____

Rhythm: _____

P wave: _____

PRI: _____

QRS: _____

Interpretation: _____

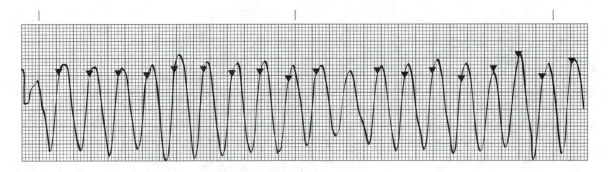

211. Rate: _____

Rhythm: _____

P wave: _____

PRI: _____

QRS: _____

Interpretation: _____

212. Rate: _____

Rhythm: _____

P wave: _____

PRI: _____

QRS: _____

Interpretation: _____

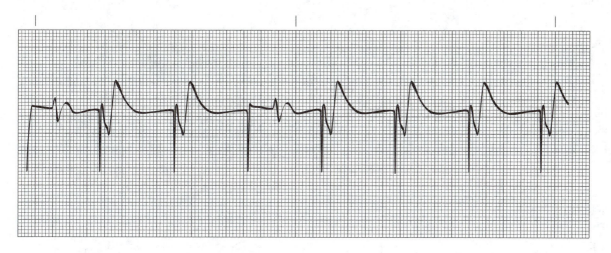

213. Rate: _____
     Rhythm: _____
     P wave: _____
     PRI: _____
     QRS: _____

     Interpretation: _____

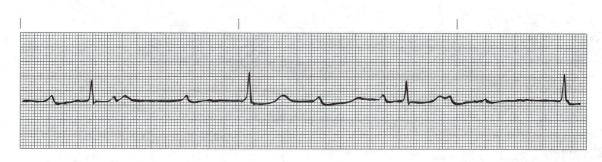

214. Rate: _____
     Rhythm: _____
     P wave: _____
     PRI: _____
     QRS: _____

     Interpretation: _____

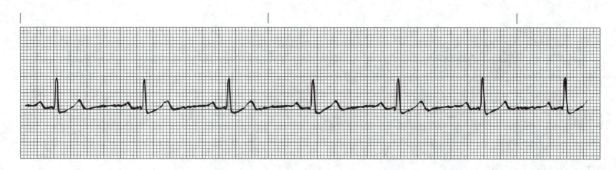

215. Rate: _____

Rhythm: _____

P Wave: _____

PRI: _____

QRS: _____

Interpretation: _____

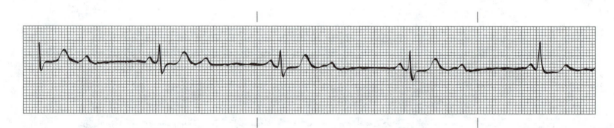

216. Rate: _____

Rhythm: _____

P wave: _____

PRI: _____

QRS: _____

Interpretation: _____

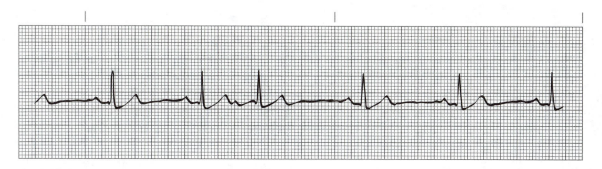

217. Rate: _____

　　 Rhythm: _____

　　 P wave: _____

　　 PRI: _____

　　 QRS: _____

　　 Interpretation: _____

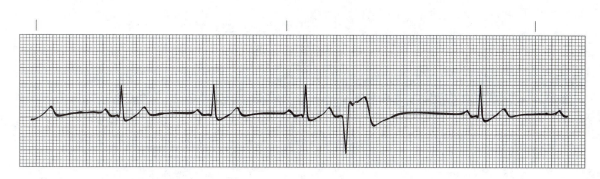

218. Rate: _____

　　 Rhythm: _____

　　 P wave: _____

　　 PRI: _____

　　 QRS: _____

　　 Interpretation: _____

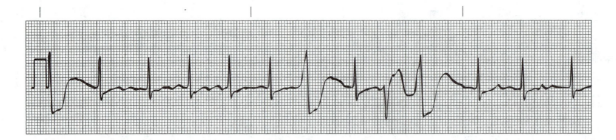

219. Rate: _____
    Rhythm: _____
    P wave: _____
    PRI: _____
    QRS: _____

    Interpretation: _____

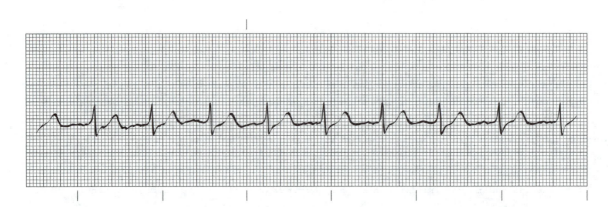

220. Rate: _____
    Rhythm: _____
    P wave: _____
    PRI: _____
    QRS: _____

    Interpretation: _____

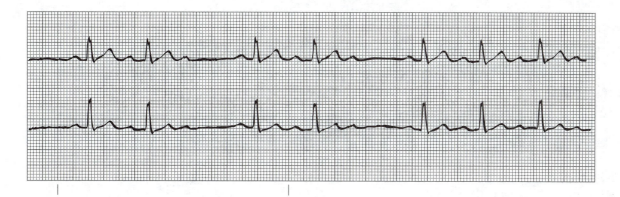

221. Rate: _____

Rhythm: _____

P wave: _____

PRI: _____

QRS: _____

Interpretation: _____

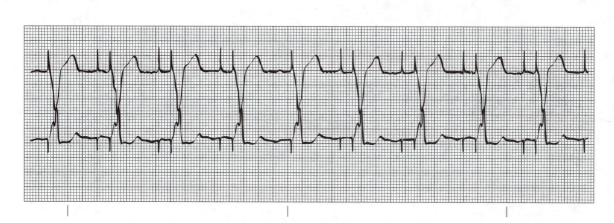

222. Rate: _____

Rhythm: _____

P wave: _____

PRI: _____

QRS: _____

Interpretation: _____

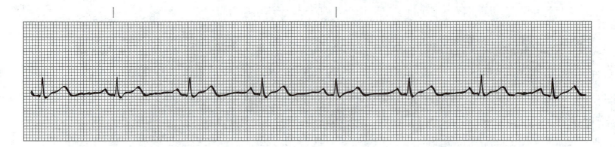

223. Rate: _____

Rhythm: _____

P wave: _____

PRI: _____

QRS: _____

Interpretation: _____

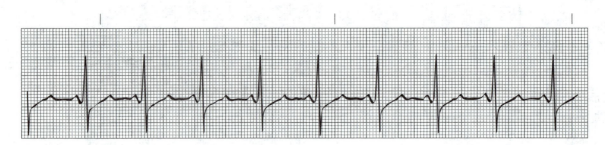

224. Rate: _____

Rhythm: _____

P wave: _____

PRI: _____

QRS: _____

Interpretation: _____

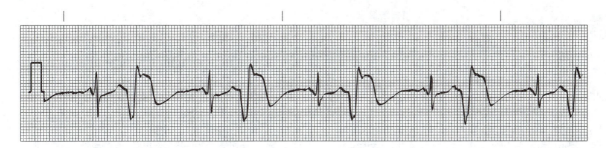

225. Rate: _____
    Rhythm: _____
    P wave: _____
    PRI: _____
    QRS: _____

    Interpretation: _____

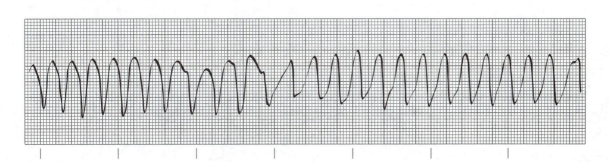

226. Rate: _____
    Rhythm: _____
    P wave: _____
    PRI: _____
    QRS: _____

    Interpretation: _____

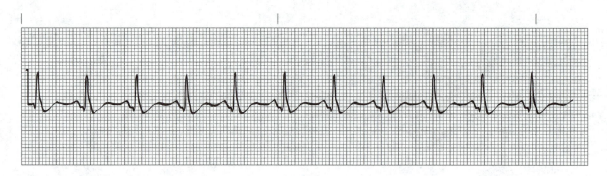

227. Rate: _____

    Rhythm: _____

    P wave: _____

    PRI: _____

    QRS: _____

    Interpretation: _____

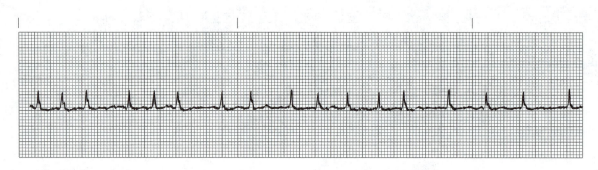

228. Rate: _____

    Rhythm: _____

    P wave: _____

    PRI: _____

    QRS: _____

    Interpretation: _____

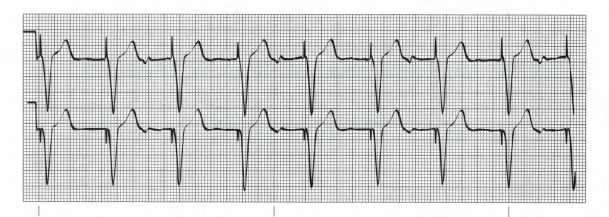

229. Rate: _____

Rhythm: _____

P wave: _____

PRI: _____

QRS: _____

Interpretation: _____

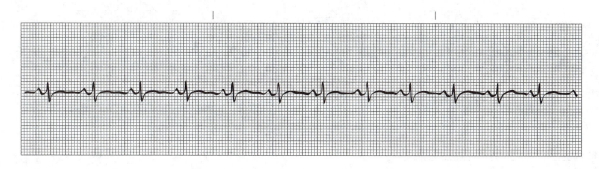

230. Rate: _____

Rhythm: _____

P wave: _____

PRI: _____

QRS: _____

Interpretation: _____

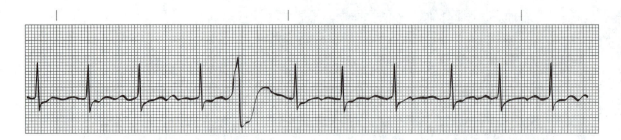

231. Rate: _____

    Rhythm: _____

    P wave: _____

    PRI: _____

    QRS: _____

    Interpretation: _____

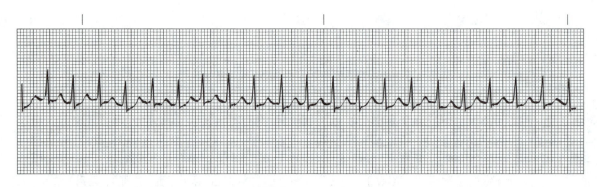

232. Rate: _____

    Rhythm: _____

    P wave: _____

    PRI: _____

    QRS: _____

    Interpretation: _____

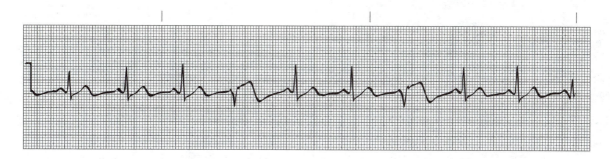

233. Rate: _____

Rhythm: _____

P wave: _____

PRI: _____

QRS: _____

Interpretation: _____

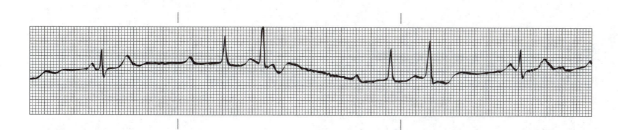

234. Rate: _____

Rhythm: _____

P wave: _____

PRI: _____

QRS: _____

Interpretation: _____

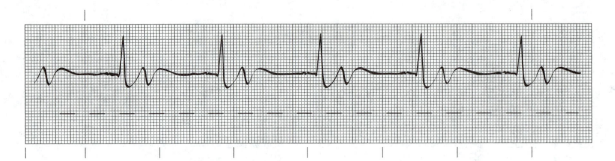

235. Rate: _____

Rhythm: _____

P wave: _____

PRI: _____

QRS: _____

Interpretation: _____

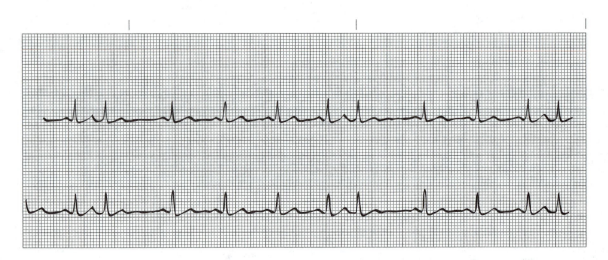

236. Rate: _____

Rhythm: _____

P wave: _____

PRI: _____

QRS: _____

Interpretation: _____

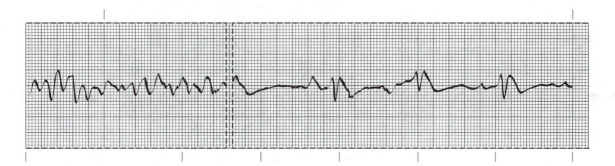

237. Rate: _____

Rhythm: _____

P wave: _____

PRI: _____

QRS: _____

Interpretation: _____

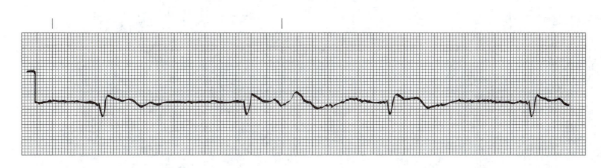

238. Rate: _____

Rhythm: _____

P wave: _____

PRI: _____

QRS: _____

Interpretation: _____

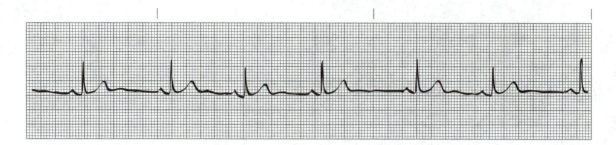

239. Rate: _____

    Rhythm: _____

    P wave: _____

    PRI: _____

    QRS: _____

    Interpretation: _____

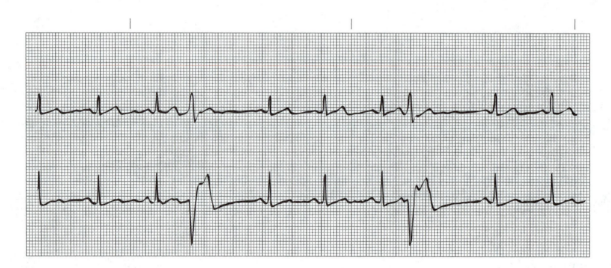

240. Rate: _____

    Rhythm: _____

    P wave: _____

    PRI: _____

    QRS: _____

    Interpretation: _____

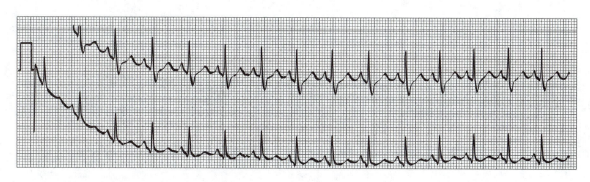

241. Rate: _____

     Rhythm: _____

     P wave: _____

     PRI: _____

     QRS: _____

     Interpretation: _____

242. Rate: _____

     Rhythm: _____

     P wave: _____

     PRI: _____

     QRS: _____

     Interpretation: _____

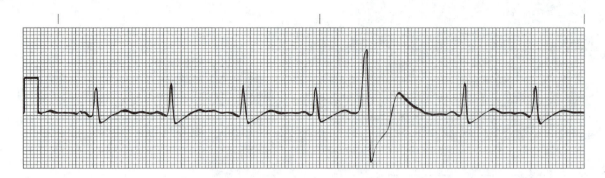

243. Rate: _____

Rhythm: _____

P wave: _____

PRI: _____

QRS: _____

Interpretation: _____

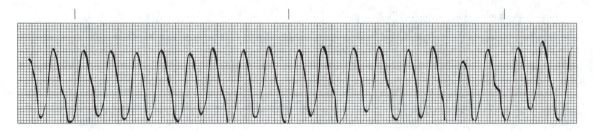

244. Rate: _____

Rhythm: _____

P wave: _____

PRI: _____

QRS: _____

Interpretation: _____

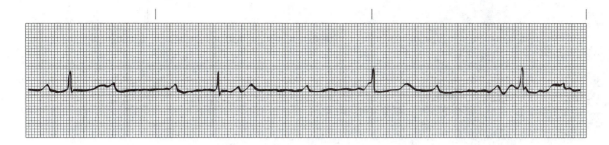

245. Rate: _____
     Rhythm: _____
     P wave: _____
     PRI: _____
     QRS: _____

     Interpretation: _____

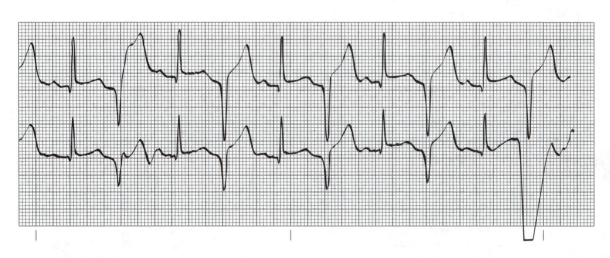

246. Rate: _____
     Rhythm: _____
     P wave: _____
     PRI: _____
     QRS: _____

     Interpretation: _____

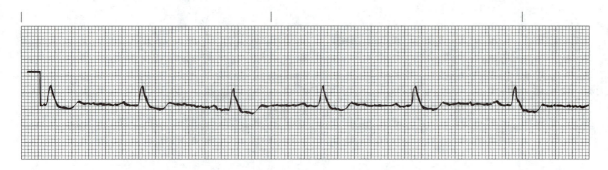

247. Rate: _____

     Rhythm: _____

     P wave: _____

     PRI: _____

     QRS: _____

     Interpretation: _____

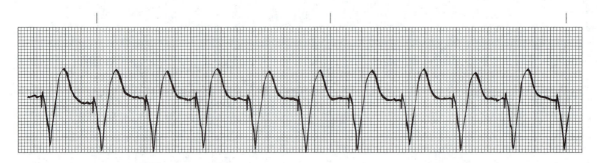

248. Rate: _____

     Rhythm: _____

     P wave: _____

     PRI: _____

     QRS: _____

     Interpretation: _____

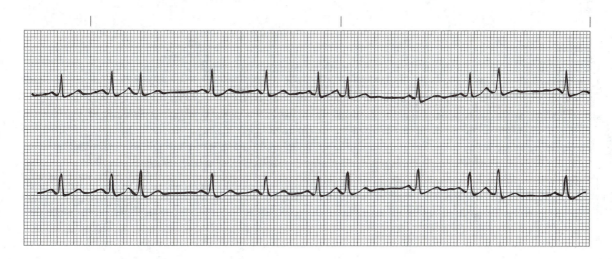

249. Rate: _____

   Rhythm: _____

   P wave: _____

   PRI: _____

   QRS: _____

   Interpretation: _____

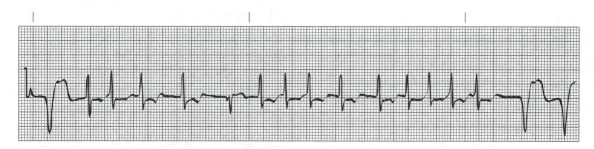

250. Rate: _____

   Rhythm: _____

   P wave: _____

   PRI: _____

   QRS: _____

   Interpretation: _____

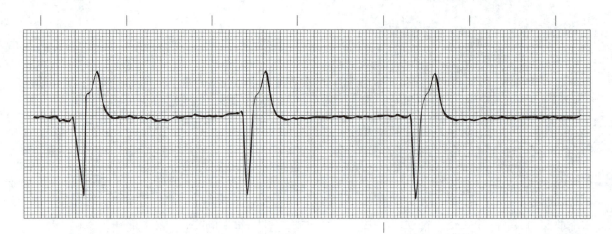

251. Rate: _____

    Rhythm: _____

    P wave: _____

    PRI: _____

    QRS: _____

    Interpretation: _____

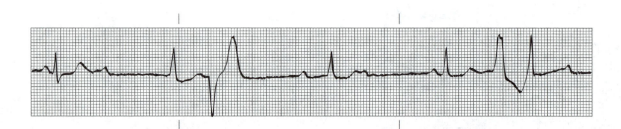

252. Rate: _____

    Rhythm: _____

    P wave: _____

    PRI: _____

    QRS: _____

    Interpretation: _____

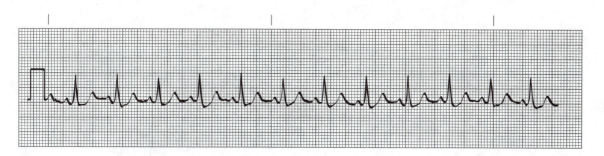

253. Rate: _____

    Rhythm: _____

    P wave: _____

    PRI: _____

    QRS: _____

    Interpretation: _____

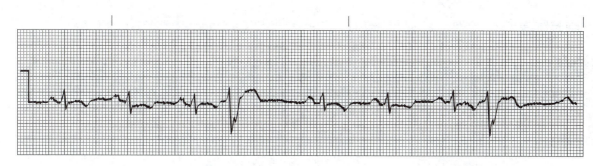

254. Rate: _____

    Rhythm: _____

    P wave: _____

    PRI: _____

    QRS: _____

    Interpretation: _____

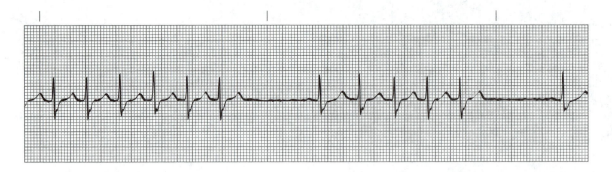

255. Rate: _____

  Rhythm: _____

  P wave: _____

  PRI: _____

  QRS: _____

  Interpretation: _____

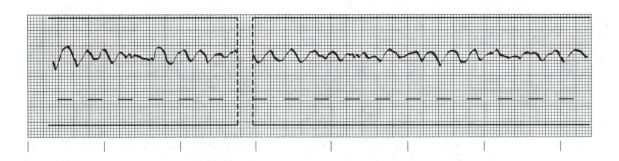

256. Rate: _____

  Rhythm: _____

  P wave: _____

  PRI: _____

  QRS: _____

  Interpretation: _____

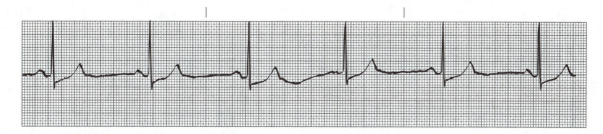

257. Rate: _____

    Rhythm: _____

    P wave: _____

    PRI: _____

    QRS: _____

    Interpretation: _____

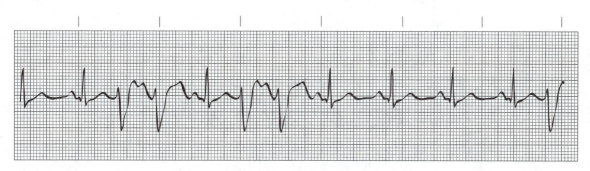

258. Rate: _____

    Rhythm: _____

    P wave: _____

    PRI: _____

    QRS: _____

    Interpretation: _____

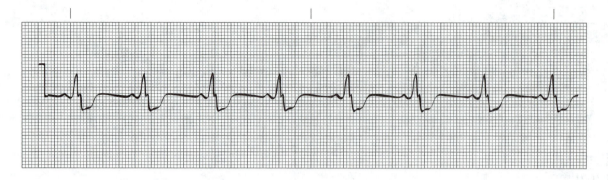

259. Rate: _____

Rhythm: _____

P wave: _____

PRI: _____

QRS: _____

Interpretation: _____

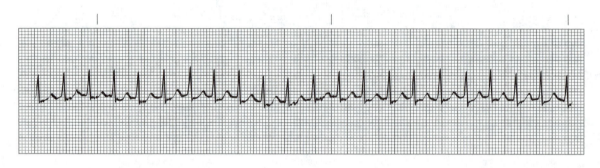

260. Rate: _____

Rhythm: _____

P wave: _____

PRI: _____

QRS: _____

Interpretation: _____

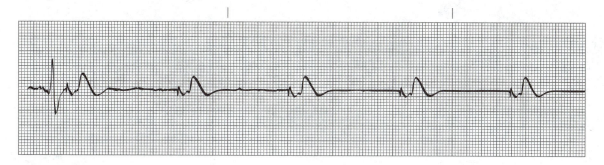

261. Rate: _____

     Rhythm: _____

     P wave: _____

     PRI: _____

     QRS: _____

     Interpretation: _____

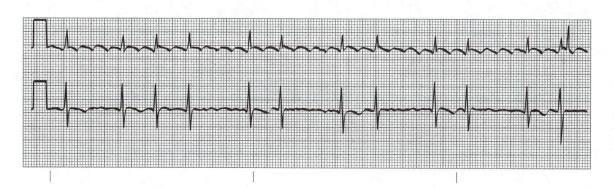

262. Rate: _____

     Rhythm: _____

     P wave: _____

     PRI: _____

     QRS: _____

     Interpretation: _____

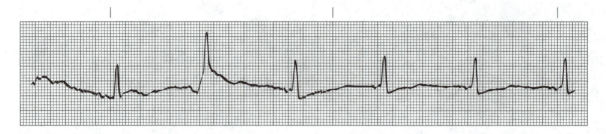

263. Rate: _____

Rhythm: _____

P wave: _____

PRI: _____

QRS: _____

Interpretation: _____

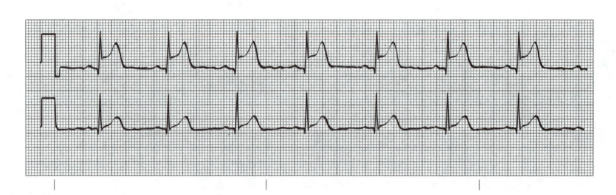

264. Rate: _____

Rhythm: _____

P wave: _____

PRI: _____

QRS: _____

Interpretation: _____

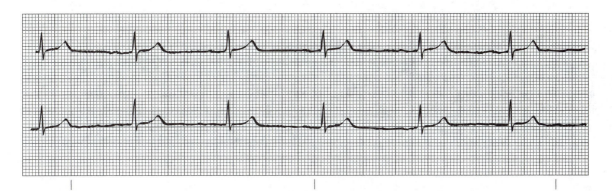

265. Rate: _____

   Rhythm: _____

   P wave: _____

   PRI: _____

   QRS: _____

   Interpretation: _____

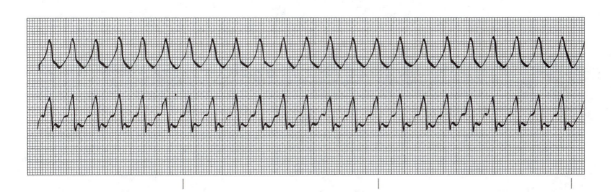

266. Rate: _____

   Rhythm: _____

   P wave: _____

   PRI: _____

   QRS: _____

   Interpretation: _____

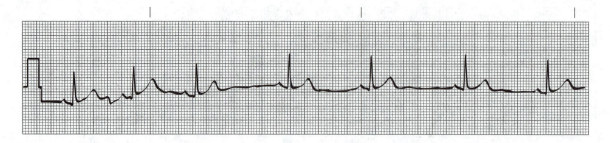

267. Rate: _____

Rhythm: _____

P wave: _____

PRI: _____

QRS: _____

Interpretation: _____

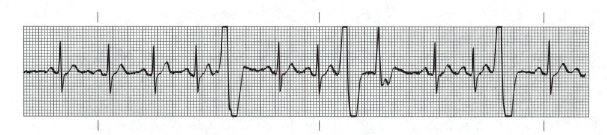

268. Rate: _____

Rhythm: _____

P wave: _____

PRI: _____

QRS: _____

Interpretation: _____

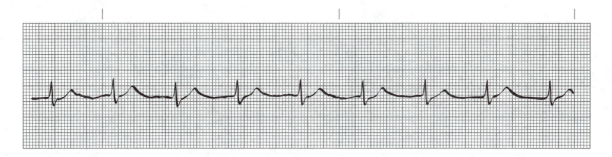

269. Rate: _____
     Rhythm: _____
     P wave: _____
     PRI: _____
     QRS: _____

     Interpretation: _____

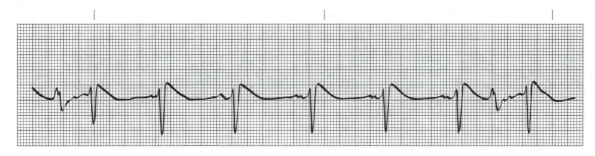

270. Rate: _____
     Rhythm: _____
     P wave: _____
     PRI: _____
     QRS: _____

     Interpretation: _____

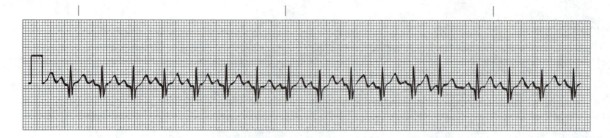

271. Rate: _____

    Rhythm: _____

    P wave: _____

    PRI: _____

    QRS: _____

    Interpretation: _____

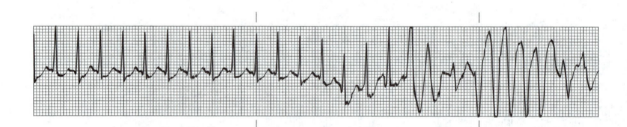

272. Rate: _____

    Rhythm: _____

    P wave: _____

    PRI: _____

    QRS: _____

    Interpretation: _____

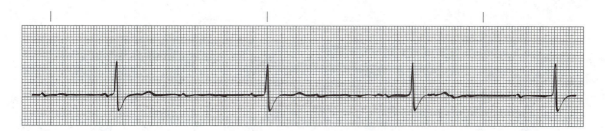

273. Rate: _____
    Rhythm: _____
    P wave: _____
    PRI: _____
    QRS: _____

    Interpretation: _____

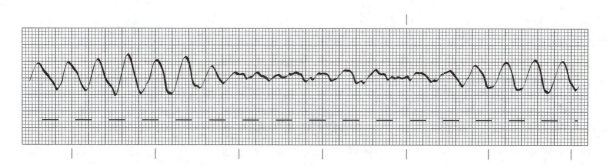

274. Rate: _____
    Rhythm: _____
    P wave: _____
    PRI: _____
    QRS: _____

    Interpretation: _____

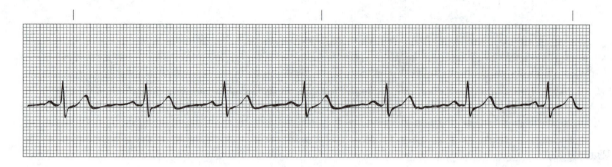

275. Rate: _____

Rhythm: _____

P wave: _____

PRI: _____

QRS: _____

Interpretation: _____

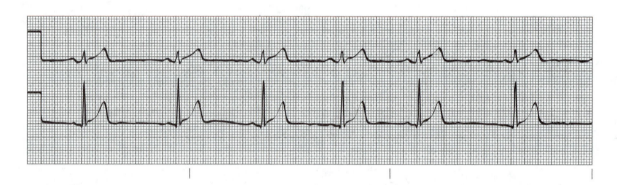

276. Rate: _____

Rhythm: _____

P wave: _____

PRI: _____

QRS: _____

Interpretation: _____

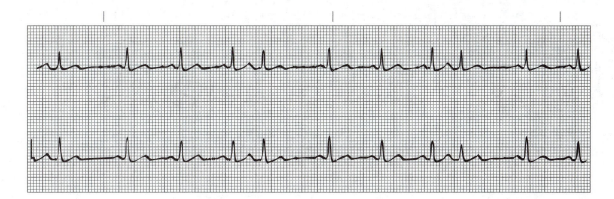

277. Rate: _____

Rhythm: _____

P wave: _____

PRI: _____

QRS: _____

Interpretation: _____

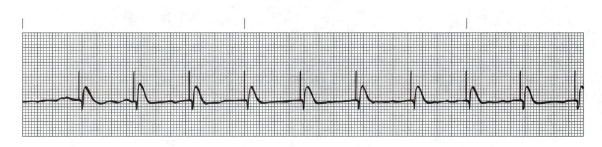

278. Rate: _____

Rhythm: _____

P wave: _____

PRI: _____

QRS: _____

Interpretation: _____

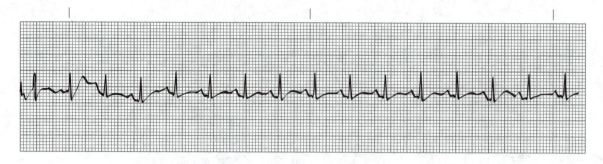

279. Rate: _____

Rhythm: _____

P wave: _____

PRI: _____

QRS: _____

Interpretation: _____

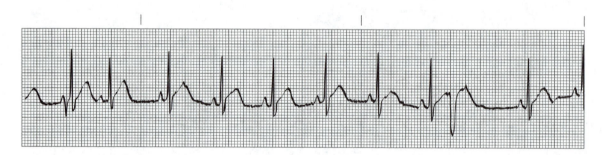

280. Rate: _____

Rhythm: _____

P wave: _____

PRI: _____

QRS: _____

Interpretation: _____

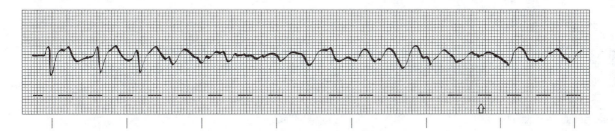

281. Rate: _____

    Rhythm: _____

    P wave: _____

    PRI: _____

    QRS: _____

    Interpretation: _____

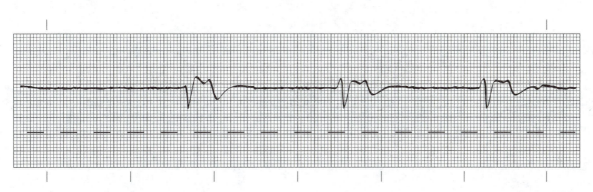

282. Rate: _____

    Rhythm: _____

    P wave: _____

    PRI: _____

    QRS: _____

    Interpretation: _____

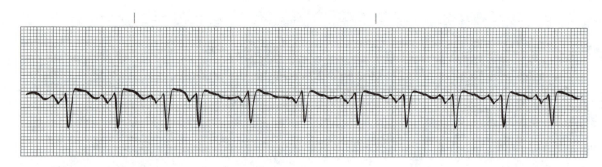

283. Rate: _____

   Rhythm: _____

   P wave: _____

   PRI: _____

   QRS: _____

   Interpretation: _____

284. Rate: _____

   Rhythm: _____

   P wave: _____

   PRI: _____

   QRS: _____

   Interpretation: _____

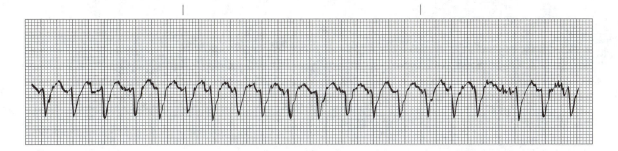

285. Rate: _____

Rhythm: _____

P wave: _____

PRI: _____

QRS: _____

Interpretation: _____

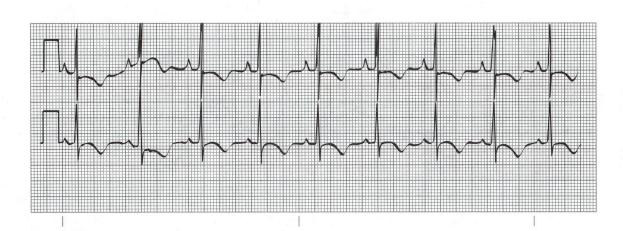

286. Rate: _____

Rhythm: _____

P wave: _____

PRI: _____

QRS: _____

Interpretation: _____

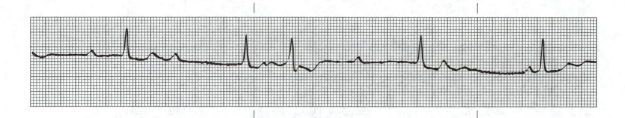

287. Rate: _____

Rhythm: _____

P wave: _____

PRI: _____

QRS: _____

Interpretation: _____

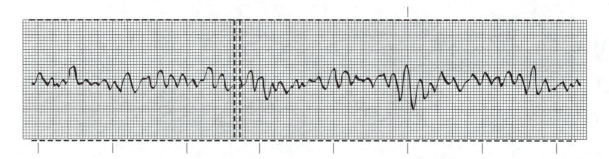

288. Rate: _____

Rhythm: _____

P wave: _____

PRI: _____

QRS: _____

Interpretation: _____

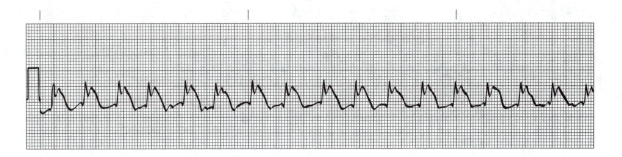

289. Rate: _____
    Rhythm: _____
    P wave: _____
    PRI: _____
    QRS: _____

    Interpretation: _____

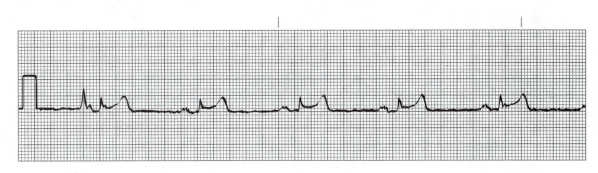

290. Rate: _____
    Rhythm: _____
    P wave: _____
    PRI: _____
    QRS: _____

    Interpretation: _____

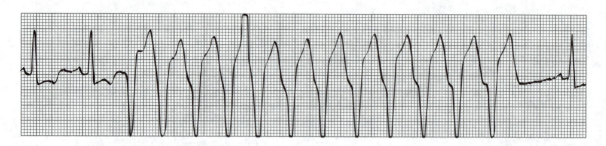

291. Rate: _____

    Rhythm: _____

    P wave: _____

    PRI: _____

    QRS: _____

    Interpretation: _____

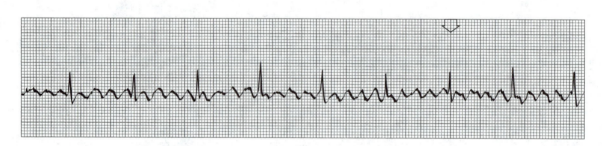

292. Rate: _____

    Rhythm: _____

    P wave: _____

    PRI: _____

    QRS: _____

    Interpretation: _____

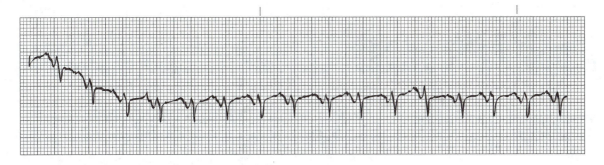

293. Rate: _____

     Rhythm: _____

     P wave: _____

     PRI: _____

     QRS: _____

     Interpretation: _____

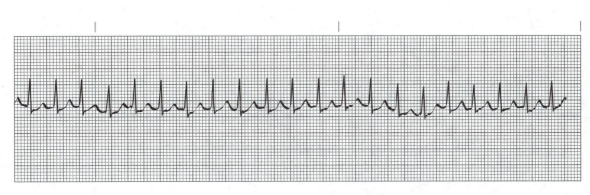

294. Rate: _____

     Rhythm: _____

     P wave: _____

     PRI: _____

     QRS: _____

     Interpretation: _____

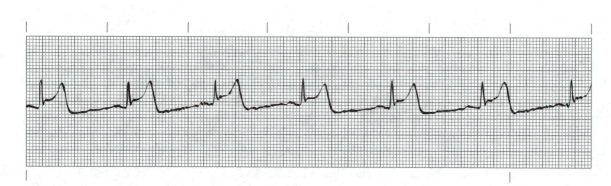

295. Rate: _____

Rhythm: _____

P wave: _____

PRI: _____

QRS: _____

Interpretation: _____

296. Rate: _____

Rhythm: _____

P wave: _____

PRI: _____

QRS: _____

Interpretation: _____

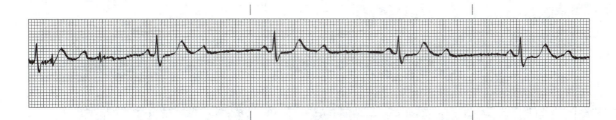

297. Rate: _____

   Rhythm: _____

   P wave: _____

   PRI: _____

   QRS: _____

   Interpretation: _____

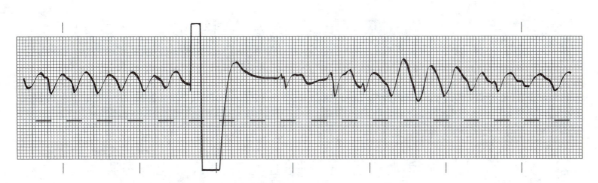

298. Rate: _____

   Rhythm: _____

   P wave: _____

   PRI: _____

   QRS: _____

   Interpretation: _____

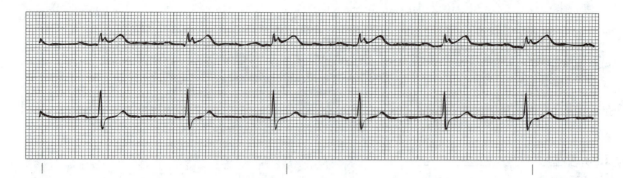

299. Rate: _____

   Rhythm: _____

   P wave: _____

   PRI: _____

   QRS: _____

   Interpretation: _____

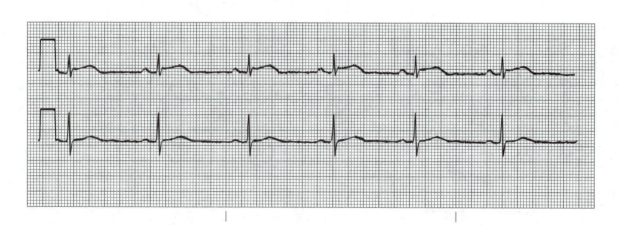

300. Rate: _____

   Rhythm: _____

   P wave: _____

   PRI: _____

   QRS: _____

   Interpretation: _____

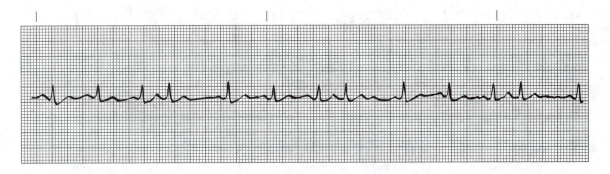

301. Rate: _____

Rhythm: _____

P wave: _____

PRI: _____

QRS: _____

Interpretation: _____

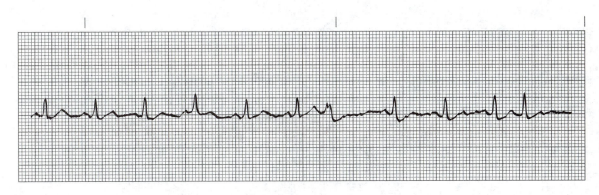

302. Rate: _____

Rhythm: _____

P wave: _____

PRI: _____

QRS: _____

Interpretation: _____

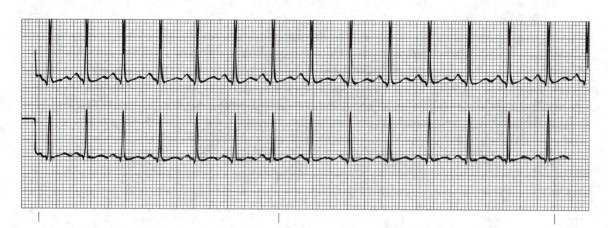

303. Rate: _____

 Rhythm: _____

 P wave: _____

 PRI: _____

 QRS: _____

 Interpretation: _____

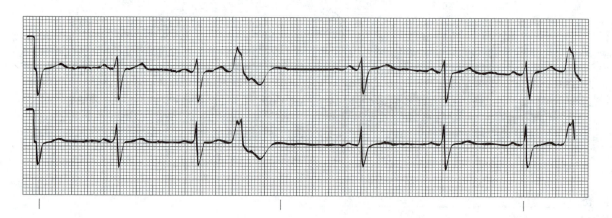

304. Rate: _____

 Rhythm: _____

 P wave: _____

 PRI: _____

 QRS: _____

 Interpretation: _____

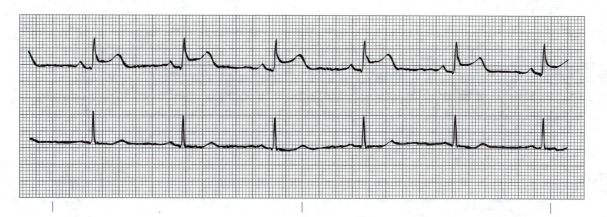

305. Rate: _____

Rhythm: _____

P wave: _____

PRI: _____

QRS: _____

Interpretation: _____

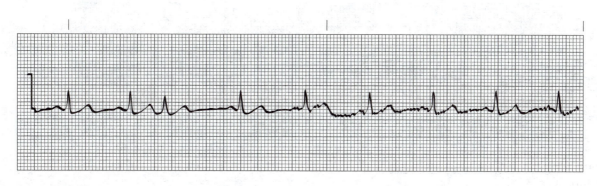

306. Rate: _____

Rhythm: _____

P wave: _____

PRI: _____

QRS: _____

Interpretation: _____

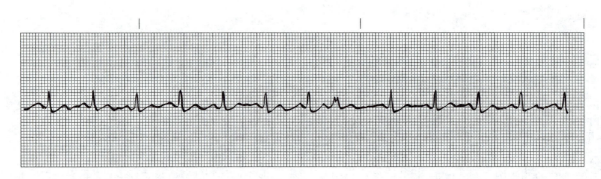

307. Rate: _____

Rhythm: _____

P wave: _____

PRI: _____

QRS: _____

Interpretation: _____

308. Rate: _____

Rhythm: _____

P wave: _____

PRI: _____

QRS: _____

Interpretation: _____

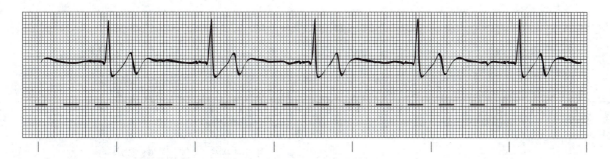

309. Rate: _____

   Rhythm: _____

   P wave: _____

   PRI: _____

   QRS: _____

   Interpretation: _____

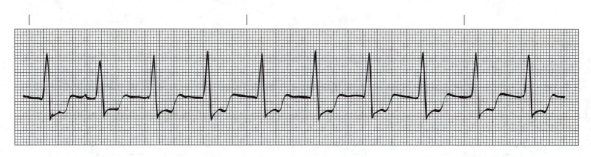

310. Rate: _____

   Rhythm: _____

   P wave: _____

   PRI: _____

   QRS: _____

   Interpretation: _____

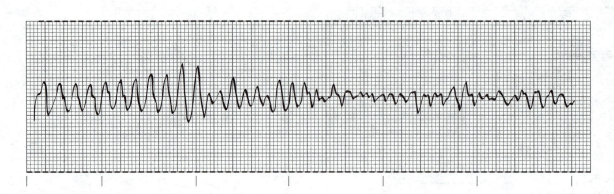

311. Rate: _____

    Rhythm: _____

    P wave: _____

    PRI: _____

    QRS: _____

    Interpretation: _____

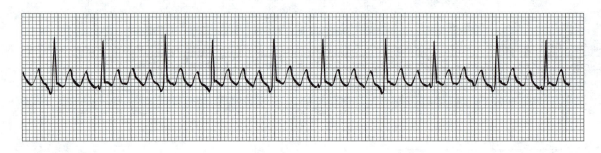

312. Rate: _____

    Rhythm: _____

    P wave: _____

    PRI: _____

    Interpretation: _____

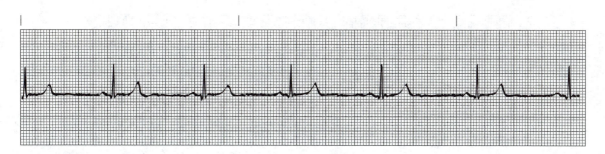

313. Rate: _____

Rhythm: _____

P wave: _____

PRI: _____

QRS: _____

Interpretation: _____

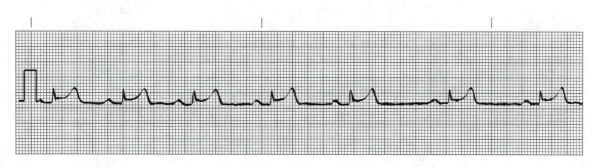

314. Rate: _____

Rhythm: _____

P wave: _____

PRI: _____

QRS: _____

Interpretation: _____

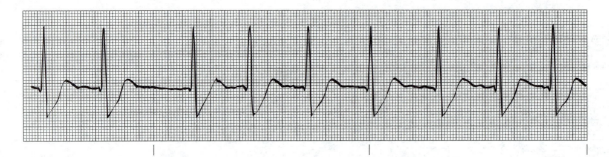

315. Rate: _____

Rhythm: _____

P wave: _____

PRI: _____

QRS: _____

Interpretation: _____

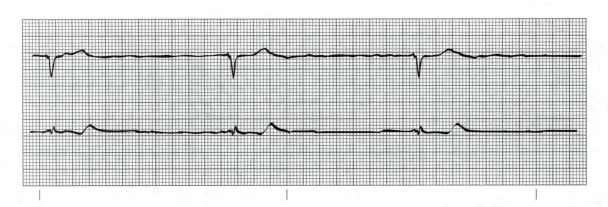

316. Rate _____

Rhythm: _____

P wave: _____

PRI: _____

QRS: _____

Interpretation: _____

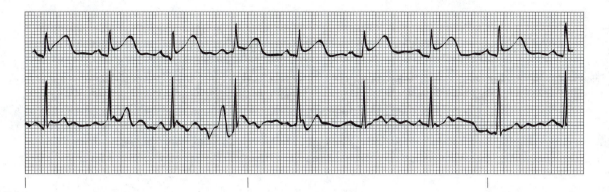

317. Rate: _____

     Rhythm: _____

     P wave: _____

     PRI: _____

     QRS: _____

     Interpretation: _____

318. Rate: _____

     Rhythm: _____

     P wave: _____

     PRI: _____

     QRS: _____

     Interpretation: _____

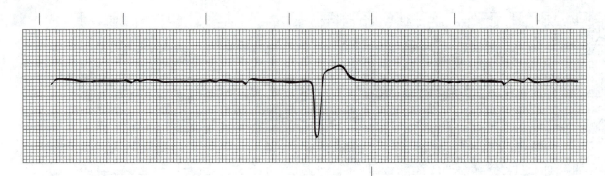

319. Rate: _____

    Rhythm: _____

    P wave: _____

    PRI: _____

    QRS: _____

    Interpretation: _____

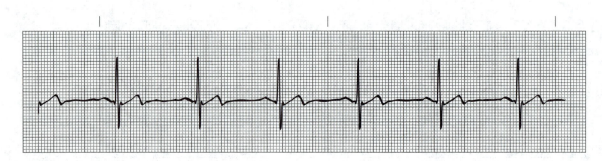

320. Rate: _____

    Rhythm: _____

    P wave: _____

    PRI: _____

    QRS: _____

    Interpretation: _____

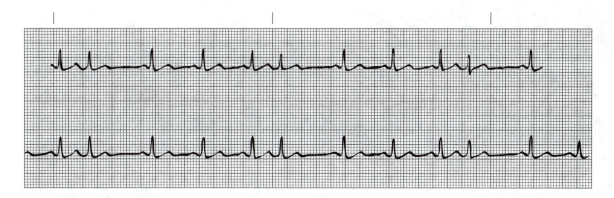

321. Rate: _____

Rhythm: _____

P wave: _____

PRI: _____

QRS: _____

Interpretation: _____

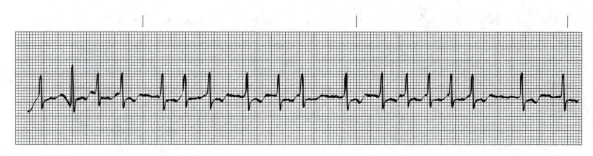

322. Rate: _____

Rhythm: _____

P wave: _____

PRI: _____

QRS: _____

Interpretation: _____

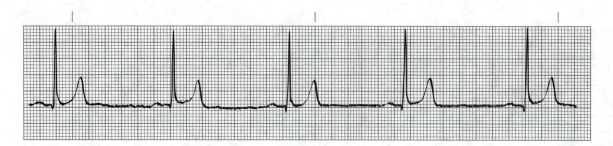

323. Rate: _____

Rhythm: _____

P wave: _____

PRI: _____

QRS: _____

Interpretation: _____

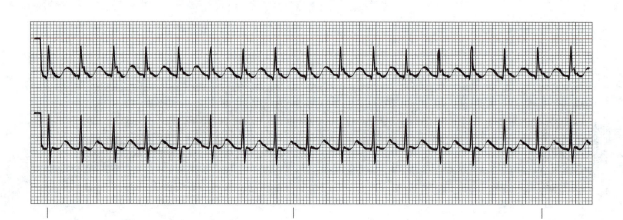

324. Rate: _____

Rhythm: _____

P wave: _____

PRI: _____

QRS: _____

Interpretation: _____

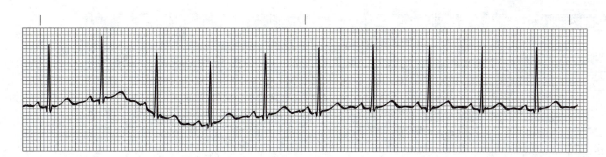

325. Rate: _____

Rhythm: _____

P wave: _____

PRI: _____

QRS: _____

Interpretation: _____

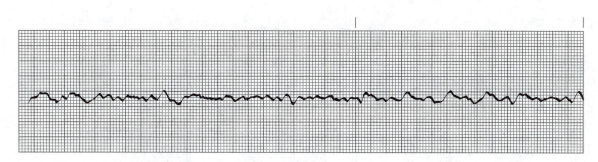

326. Rate: _____

Rhythm: _____

P wave: _____

PRI: _____

QRS: _____

Interpretation: _____

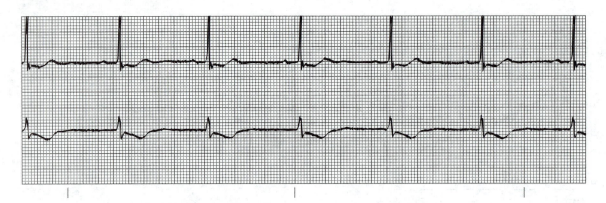

327. Rate: _____

Rhythm: _____

P wave: _____

PRI: _____

QRS: _____

Interpretation: _____

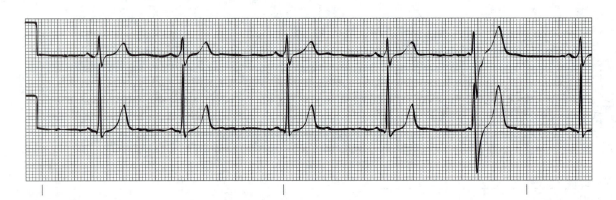

328. Rate: _____

Rhythm: _____

P wave: _____

PRI: _____

QRS: _____

Interpretation: _____

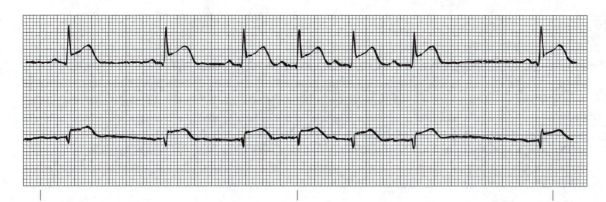

329. Rate: _____

     Rhythm: _____

     P wave: _____

     PRI: _____

     QRS: _____

     Interpretation: _____

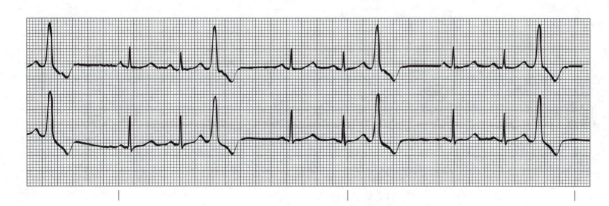

330. Rate: _____

     Rhythm: _____

     P wave: _____

     PRI: _____

     QRS: _____

     Interpretation: _____

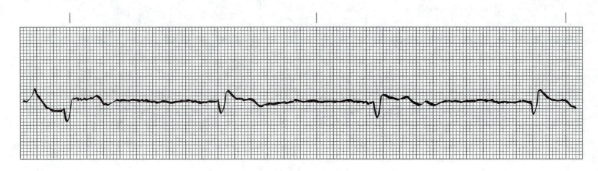

331. Rate: _____

 Rhythm: _____

 P wave: _____

 PRI: _____

 QRS: _____

 Interpretation: _____

332. Rate: _____

 Rhythm: _____

 P wave: _____

 PRI: _____

 QRS: _____

 Interpretation: _____

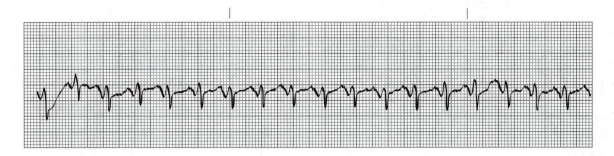

333. Rate: _____
     Rhythm: _____
     P wave: _____
     PRI: _____
     QRS: _____

     Interpretation: _____

334. Rate: _____
     Rhythm: _____
     P wave: _____
     PRI: _____
     QRS: _____

     Interpretation: _____

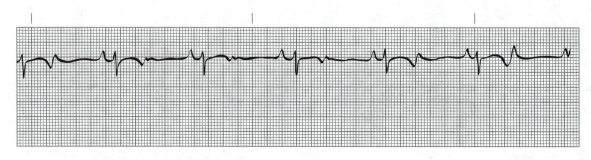

335. Rate: _____

     Rhythm: _____

     P wave: _____

     PRI: _____

     QRS: _____

     Interpretation: _____

336. Rate: _____

     Rhythm: _____

     P wave: _____

     PRI: _____

     QRS: _____

     Interpretation: _____

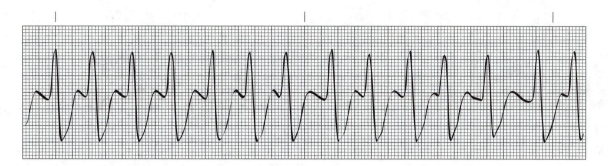

337. Rate: _____

     Rhythm: _____

     P wave: _____

     PRI: _____

     QRS: _____

     Interpretation: _____

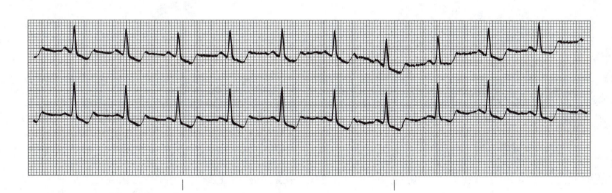

338. Rate: _____

     Rhythm: _____

     P wave: _____

     PRI: _____

     QRS: _____

     Interpretation: _____

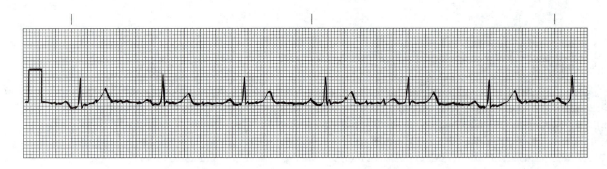

339. Rate: _____

    Rhythm: _____

    P wave: _____

    PRI: _____

    QRS: _____

    Interpretation: _____

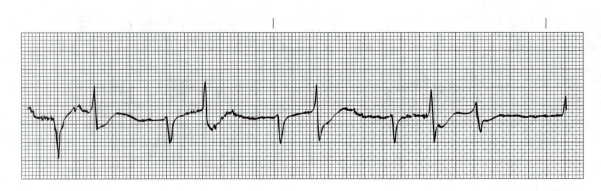

340. Rate: _____

    Rhythm: _____

    P wave: _____

    PRI: _____

    QRS: _____

    Interpretation: _____

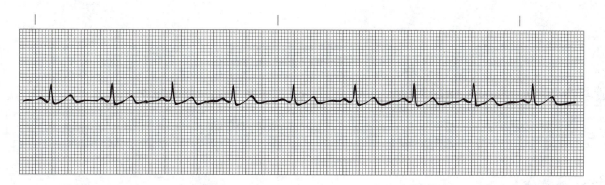

341. Rate: _____

    Rhythm: _____

    P wave: _____

    PRI: _____

    QRS: _____

    Interpretation: _____

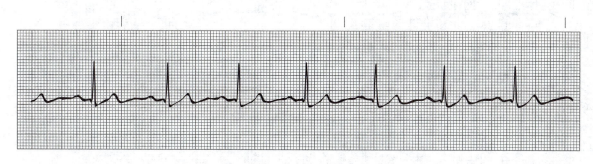

342. Rate: _____

    Rhythm: _____

    P wave: _____

    PRI: _____

    QRS: _____

    Interpretation: _____

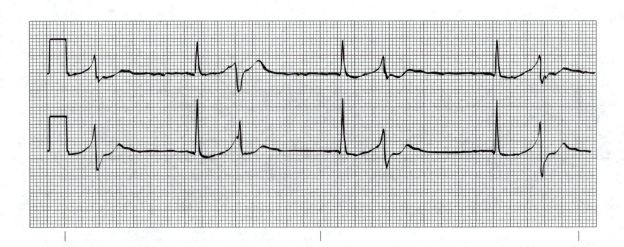

343. Rate: _____

    Rhythm: _____

    P wave: _____

    PRI: _____

    QRS: _____

    Interpretation: _____

344. Rate: _____

    Rhythm: _____

    P wave: _____

    PRI: _____

    QRS: _____

    Interpretation: _____

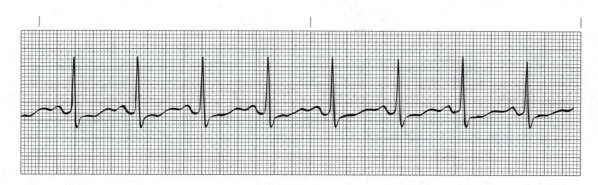

345. Rate: _____

Rhythm: _____

P wave: _____

PRI: _____

QRS: _____

Interpretation: _____

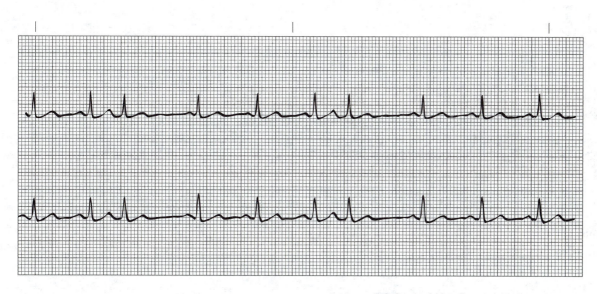

346. Rate: _____

Rhythm: _____

P wave: _____

PRI: _____

QRS: _____

Interpretation: _____

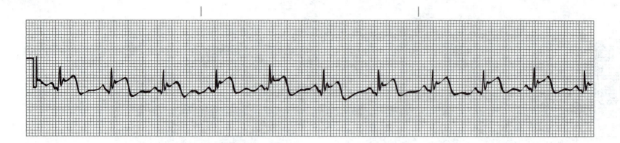

347. Rate: _____

Rhythm: _____

P wave: _____

PRI: _____

QRS: _____

Interpretation: _____

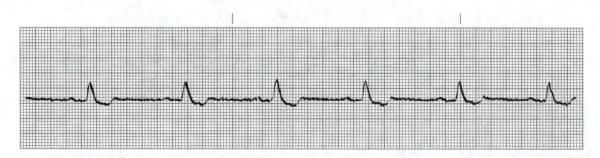

348. Rate: _____

Rhythm: _____

P wave: _____

PRI: _____

QRS: _____

Interpretation: _____

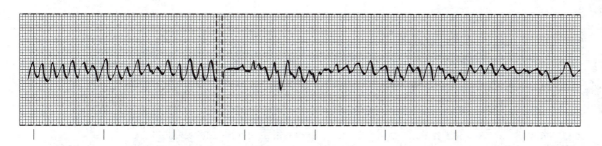

349. Rate: _____

    Rhythm: _____

    P wave: _____

    PRI: _____

    QRS: _____

    Interpretation: _____

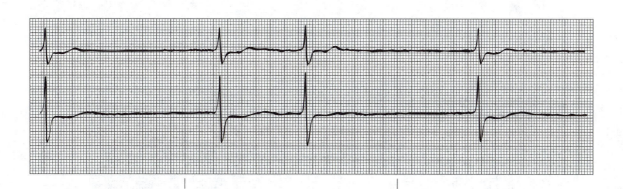

350. Rate: _____

    Rhythm: _____

    P wave: _____

    PRI: _____

    QRS: _____

    Interpretation: _____

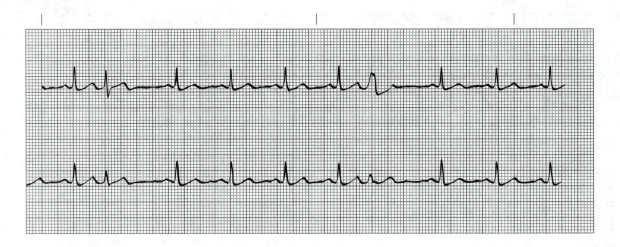

351. Rate: _____
     Rhythm: _____
     P wave: _____
     PRI: _____
     QRS: _____

     Interpretation: _____

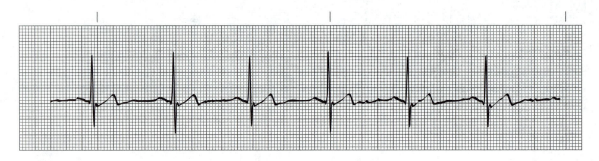

352. Rate: _____
     Rhythm: _____
     P wave: _____
     PRI: _____
     QRS: _____

     Interpretation: _____

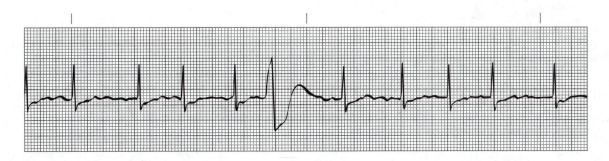

353. Rate: _____

Rhythm: _____

P wave: _____

PRI: _____

QRS: _____

Interpretation: _____

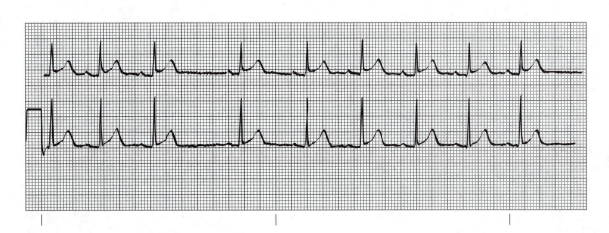

354. Rate: _____

Rhythm: _____

P wave: _____

PRI: _____

QRS: _____

Interpretation: _____

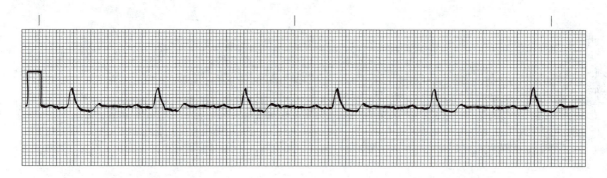

355. Rate: _____

Rhythm: _____

P wave: _____

PRI: _____

QRS: _____

Interpretation: _____

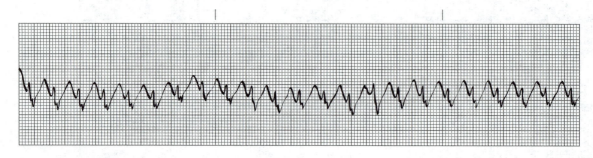

356. Rate: _____

Rhythm: _____

P wave: _____

PRI: _____

QRS: _____

Interpretation: _____

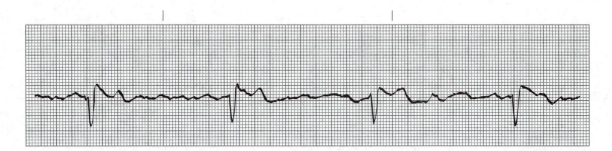

357. Rate: _____

     Rhythm: _____

     P wave: _____

     PRI: _____

     QRS: _____

     Interpretation: _____

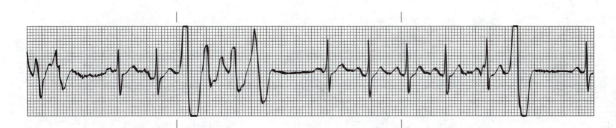

358. Rate: _____

     Rhythm: _____

     P wave: _____

     PRI: _____

     QRS: _____

     Interpretation: _____

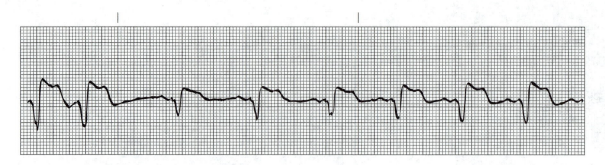

359. Rate: _____
    Rhythm: _____
    P wave: _____
    PRI: _____
    QRS: _____

    Interpretation: _____

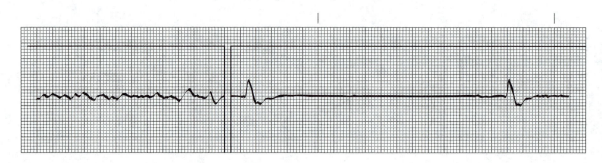

360. Rate: _____
    Rhythm: _____
    P wave: _____
    PRI: _____
    QRS: _____

    Interpretation: _____

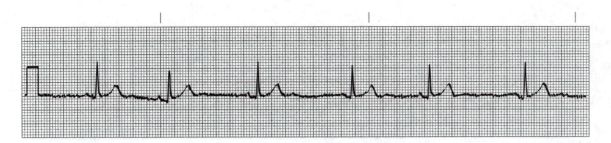

361. Rate: _____

    Rhythm: _____

    P wave: _____

    PRI: _____

    QRS: _____

    Interpretation: _____

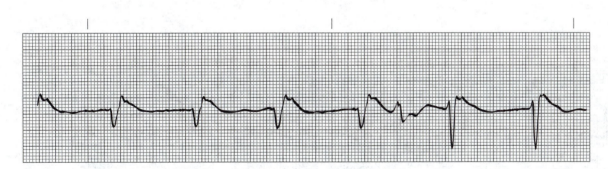

362. Rate: _____

    Rhythm: _____

    P wave: _____

    PRI: _____

    QRS: _____

    Interpretation: _____

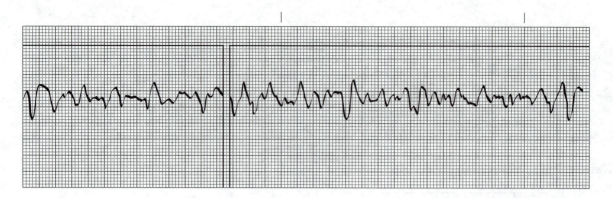

363. Rate: _____
     Rhythm: _____
     P wave: _____
     PRI: _____
     QRS: _____

     Interpretation: _____

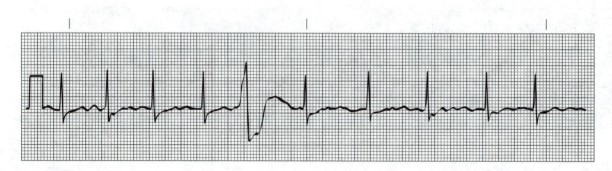

364. Rate: _____
     Rhythm: _____
     P wave: _____
     PRI: _____
     QRS: _____

     Interpretation: _____

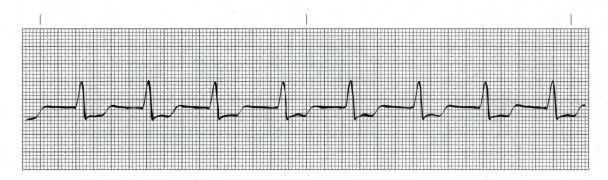

365. Rate: _____

    Rhythm: _____

    P wave: _____

    PRI: _____

    QRS: _____

    Interpretation: _____

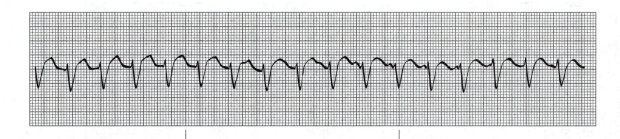

366. Rate: _____

    Rhythm: _____

    P wave: _____

    PRI: _____

    QRS: _____

    Interpretation: _____

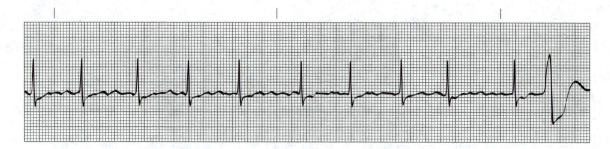

367. Rate: _____

    Rhythm: _____

    P wave: _____

    PRI: _____

    QRS: _____

    Interpretation: _____

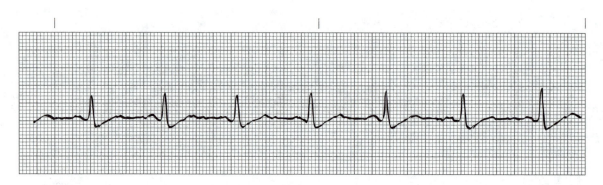

368. Rate: _____

    Rhythm: _____

    P wave: _____

    PRI: _____

    QRS: _____

    Interpretation: _____

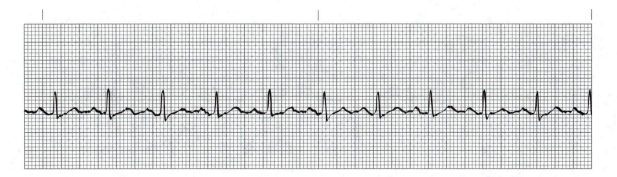

369. Rate: _____

    Rhythm: _____

    P wave: _____

    PRI: _____

    QRS: _____

    Interpretation: _____

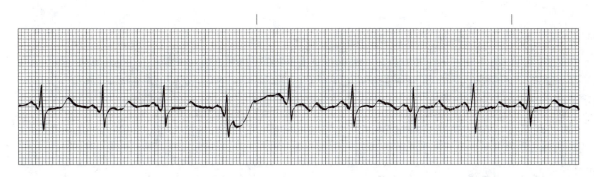

370. Rate: _____

    Rhythm: _____

    P wave: _____

    PRI: _____

    QRS: _____

    Interpretation: _____

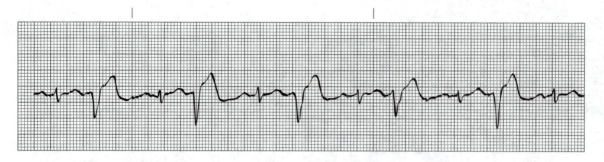

371. Rate: _____

    Rhythm: _____

    P wave: _____

    PRI: _____

    QRS: _____

    Interpretation: _____

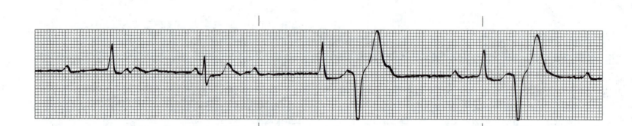

372. Rate: _____

    Rhythm: _____

    P wave: _____

    PRI: _____

    QRS: _____

    Interpretation: _____

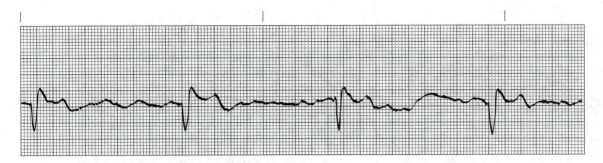

373. Rate: _____

   Rhythm: _____

   P wave: _____

   PRI: _____

   QRS: _____

   Interpretation: _____

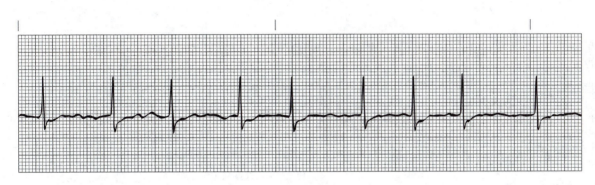

374. Rate: _____

   Rhythm: _____

   P wave: _____

   PRI: _____

   QRS: _____

   Interpretation: _____

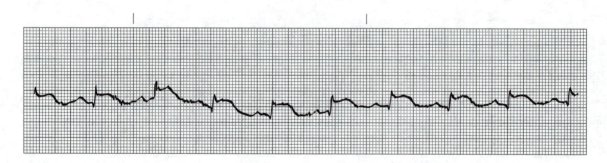

375. Rate: _____

     Rhythm: _____

     P wave: _____

     PRI: _____

     QRS: _____

     Interpretation: _____

376. Rate: _____

     Rhythm: _____

     P wave: _____

     PRI: _____

     QRS: _____

     Interpretation: _____

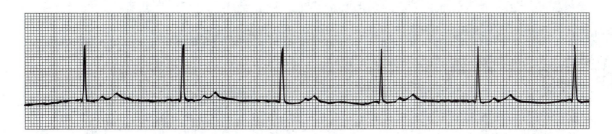

377. Rate: _____

    Rhythm: _____

    P wave: _____

    PRI: _____

    QRS: _____

    Interpretation: _____

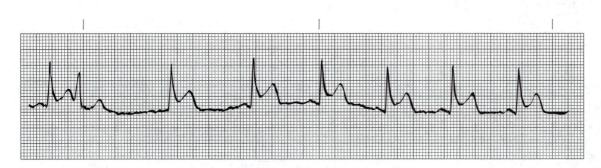

378. Rate: _____

    Rhythm: _____

    P wave: _____

    PRI: _____

    QRS: _____

    Interpretation: _____

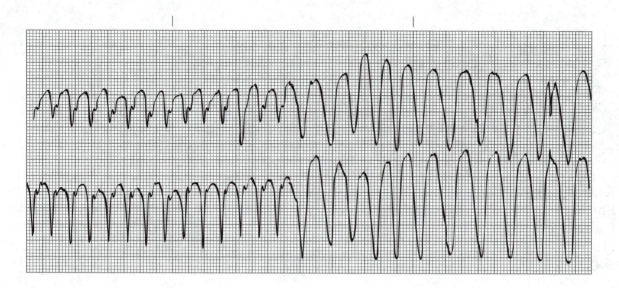

379. Rate: _____

 Rhythm: _____

 P wave: _____

 PRI: _____

 QRS: _____

 Interpretation: _____

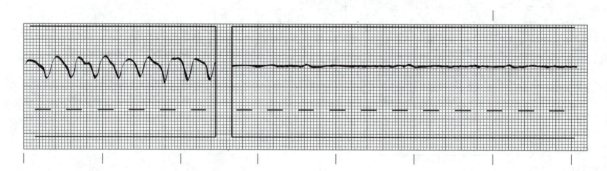

380. Rate: _____

 Rhythm: _____

 P wave: _____

 PRI: _____

 QRS: _____

 Interpretation: _____

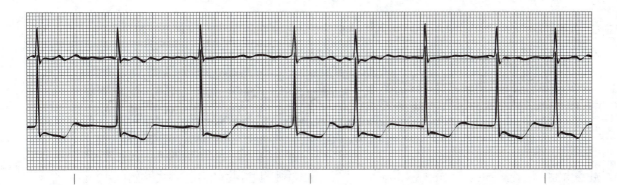

381. Rate: _____

    Rhythm: _____

    P wave: _____

    PRI: _____

    QRS: _____

    Interpretation: _____

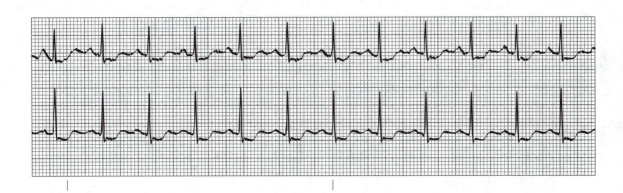

382. Rate: _____

    Rhythm: _____

    P wave: _____

    PRI: _____

    QRS: _____

    Interpretation: _____

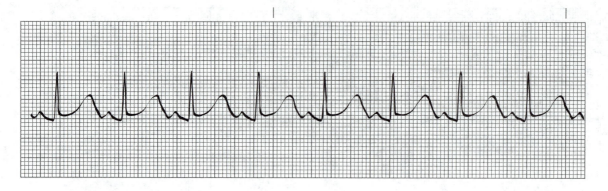

383. Rate: _____

     Rhythm: _____

     P wave: _____

     PRI: _____

     QRS: _____

     Interpretation: _____

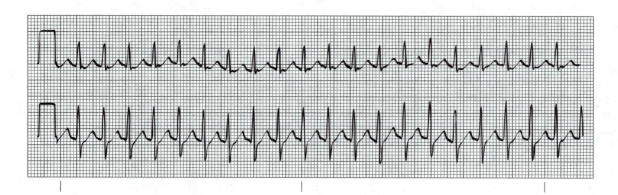

384. Rate: _____

     Rhythm: _____

     P wave: _____

     PRI: _____

     QRS: _____

     Interpretation: _____

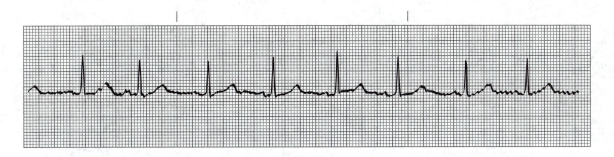

385. Rate: _____

    Rhythm: _____

    P wave: _____

    PRI: _____

    QRS: _____

    Interpretation: _____

386. Rate: _____

    Rhythm: _____

    P wave: _____

    PRI: _____

    QRS: _____

    Interpretation: _____

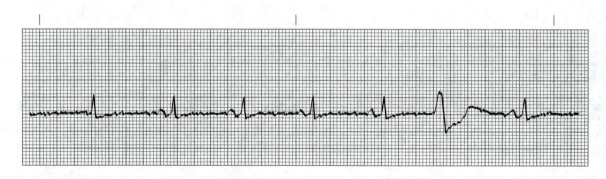

387. Rate: _____

     Rhythm: _____

     P wave: _____

     PRI: _____

     QRS: _____

     Interpretation: _____

388. Rate: _____

     Rhythm: _____

     P wave: _____

     PRI: _____

     QRS: _____

     Interpretation: _____

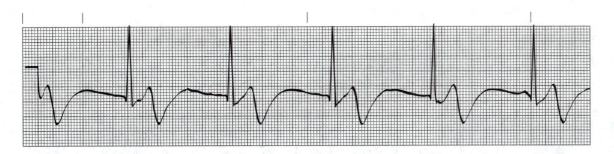

389. Rate: _____

Rhythm: _____

P wave: _____

PRI: _____

QRS: _____

Interpretation: _____

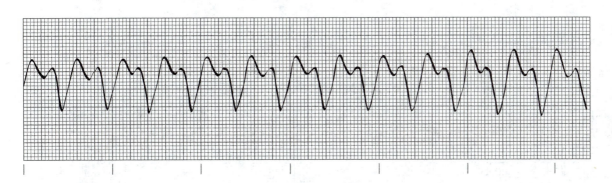

390. Rate: _____

Rhythm: _____

P wave: _____

PRI: _____

QRS: _____

Interpretation: _____

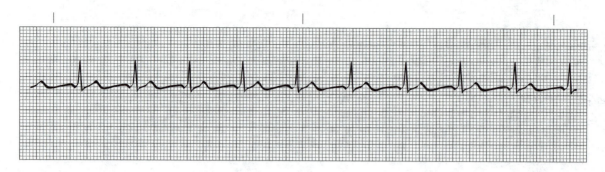

391. Rate: _____
     Rhythm: _____
     P wave: _____
     PRI: _____
     QRS: _____

     Interpretation: _____

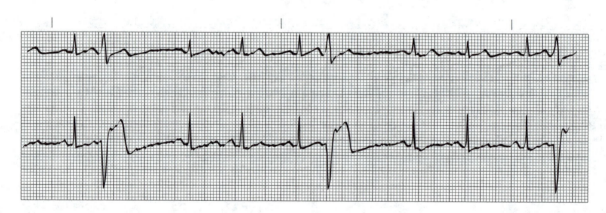

392. Rate: _____
     Rhythm: _____
     P wave: _____
     PRI: _____
     QRS: _____

     Interpretation: _____

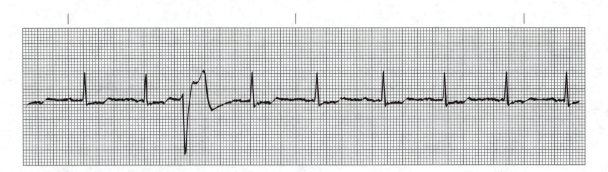

393. Rate: _____

    Rhythm: _____

    P wave: _____

    PRI: _____

    QRS: _____

    Interpretation: _____

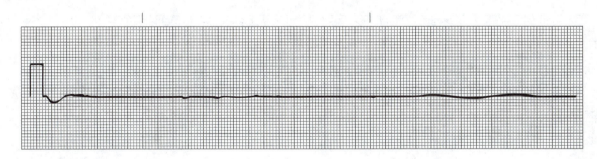

394. Rate: _____

    Rhythm: _____

    P wave: _____

    PRI: _____

    QRS: _____

    Interpretation: _____

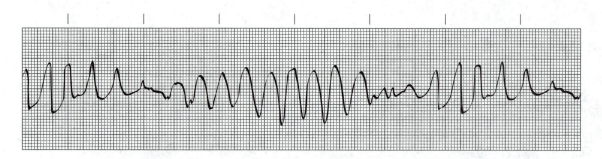

395. Rate: _____

    Rhythm: _____

    P wave: _____

    PRI: _____

    QRS: _____

    Interpretation: _____

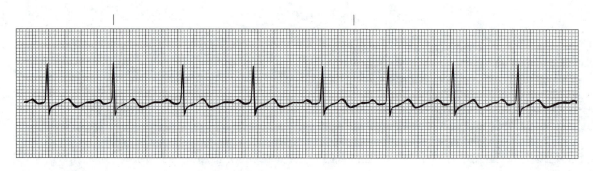

396. Rate: _____

    Rhythm: _____

    P wave: _____

    PRI: _____

    QRS: _____

    Interpretation: _____

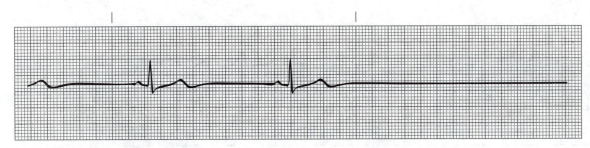

397. Rate: _____

    Rhythm: _____

    P wave: _____

    PRI: _____

    QRS: _____

    Interpretation: _____

398. Rate: _____

    Rhythm: _____

    P wave: _____

    PRI: _____

    QRS: _____

    Interpretation: _____

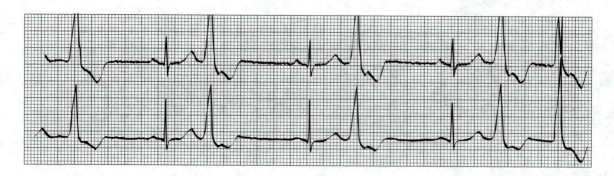

399. Rate: _____

     Rhythm: _____

     P wave: _____

     PRI: _____

     QRS: _____

     Interpretation: _____

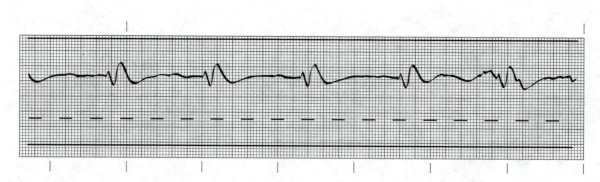

400. Rate: _____

     Rhythm: _____

     P wave: _____

     PRI: _____

     QRS: _____

     Interpretation: _____

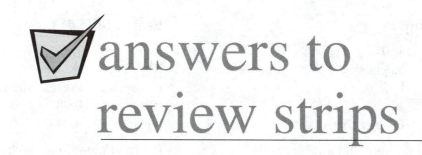 answers to
review strips

Review Strip #1

Rate: 90
Rhythm: Irregular
P wave: Present and upright
PRI: 0.12
QRS: 0.04

Interpretation: Sinus rhythm with a PVC

Review Strip #2

Rate: 60
Rhythm: Regular
P wave: Present and notched
PRI: 0.24
QRS: 0.04

Interpretation: First-degree heart block

Review Strip #3

Rate: 180
Rhythm: Irregular
P wave: I
PRI: A
QRS: 0.08

Interpretation: Atrial fibrillation with runs of ventricular tachycardia

Review Strip #4

Rate: 130
Rhythm: Irregular
P wave: A

PRI: A
QRS: 0.04

Interpretation: Atrial fibrillation

Review Strip #5

Rate: 90
Rhythm: Regular
P wave: Present and upright
PRI: 0.20
QRS: 0.12

Interpretation: Normal sinus rhythm with ST segment elevation

Review Strip #6

Rate: 60
Rhythm: Regular
P wave: Present and upright
PRI: 0.24
QRS: 0.04

Interpretation: Sinus rhythm with first-degree block

Review Strip #7

Rate: 120
Rhythm: Regular
P wave: Present and upright
PRI: 0.16
QRS: 0.04

Interpretation: Sinus tachycardia with ST segment elevation

Review Strip #8

Rate:	150
Rhythm:	Regular
P waves:	I
PRI:	A
QRS:	Greater than 0.12

Interpretation: Ventricular tachycardia

Review Strip #9

Rate:	60
Rhythm:	Regular
P wave:	Present and upright
PRI:	0.12
QRS:	0.08

Interpretation: Normal sinus rhythm

Review Strip #10

Rate:	140
Rhythm:	Irregular
P wave:	I
PRI:	A
QRS:	0.08

Interpretation: Supraventricular tachycardia (SVT) with a run of ventricular tachycardia

Review Strip #11

Rate:	90
Rhythm:	Irregular
P wave:	Present and upright
PRI:	0.20
QRS:	0.06

Interpretation: Sinus rhythm with a Premature Ventricular Complex (PVC)

Review Strip #12

Rate:	100
Rhythm:	Irregular
P wave:	I
PRI:	A
QRS:	0.06

Interpretation: Atrial fibrillation

Review Strip #13

Rate:	130
Rhythm:	Regular
P wave:	Present and upright
PRI:	0.08
QRS:	0.04

Interpretation: Sinus tachycardia

Review Strip #14

Rate:	50
Rhythm:	Irregular
P wave:	Present and upright
PRI:	0.20
QRS:	0.08

Interpretation: Sinus bradycardia with a Premature Atrial Complex (PAC)

Review Strip #15

Rate:	0
Rhythm:	A
P waves:	A
PRI:	A
QRS:	A

Interpretation: Fine ventricular fibrillation

Review Strip #16

Rate:	110
Rhythm:	Irregular
P wave:	I
PRI:	A
QRS:	0.04

Interpretation: Atrial fibrillation

Review Strip #17

Rate:	90
Rhythm:	Regular
P wave:	Present and upright
PRI:	0.16
QRS:	0.08

Interpretation: Sinus rhythm with artifact

Review Strip #18

Rate: 90
Rhythm: Irregular
P wave: Present and upright
PRI: 0.22
QRS: 0.08

Interpretation: First-degree heart block with a PVC

Review Strip #19

Rate: 90
Rhythm: Regular
P wave: Present and upright
PRI: 0.20
QRS: 0.08

Interpretation: Normal sinus rhythm with ST segment elevation (3 mm)

Review Strip #20

Rate: A
Rhythm: I
P wave: I
PRI: I
QRS: I

Interpretation: Fine ventricular fibrillation

Review Strip #21

Rate: 80
Rhythm: Irregular
P wave: Present and upright
PRI: 0.16
QRS: 0.08

Interpretation: Sinus rhythm with run of bigeminy PVCs

Review Strip #22

Rate: 120
Rhythm: Regular
P wave: Present and upright
PRI: 0.16
QRS: 0.04

Interpretation: Sinus tachycardia

Review Strip #23

Rate: 150
Rhythm: Slightly Irregular
P wave: Present and upright
PRI: 0.24
QRS: 0.04

Interpretation: Sinus tachycardia with first-degree block; postshock

Review Strip #24

Rate: 110
Rhythm: Irregular
P wave: I
PRI: A
QRS: 0.08

Interpretation: Atrial fibrillation

Review Strip #25

Rate: 160
Rhythm: Irregular
P wave: A
PRI: I
QRS: 0.08

Interpretation: Atrial fibrillation with rapid ventricular response

Review Strip #26

Rate: 40
Rhythm: Regular
P wave: Present and upright
PRI: 0.20
QRS: 0.08

Interpretation: Sinus bradycardia

Review Strip #27

Rate: 0
Rhythm: Irregular
P wave: A
PRI: 0
QRS: 0

Interpretation: Coarse ventricular fibrillation

Review Strip #28

Rate: 30
Rhythm: Regular
P wave: Present and inverted
PRI: 0.32
QRS: 0.10

Interpretation: Second-degree heart block; Mobitz type II; 2:1 block

Review Strip #29

Rate: 40
Rhythm: Regular
P wave: Present and inverted
PRI: 0.10
QRS: 0.04

Interpretation: Junctional bradycardia

Review Strip #30

Rate: 100
Rhythm: Regular
P wave: Absent or may be buried in the QRS
PRI: A
QRS: 0.08

Interpretation: Junctional tachycardia

Review Strip #31

Rate: 150
Rhythm: Regular
P wave: Present and upright
PRI: 0.16
QRS: 0.04

Interpretation: Sinus tachycardia

Review Strip #32

Rate: 70
Rhythm: Regular
P wave: Replaced with flutter waves
PRI: A
QRS: 0.04

Interpretation: Atrial flutter

Review Strip #33

Rate: 30
Rhythm: Regular
P wave: Present and upright
PRI: 0.16
QRS: 0.04

Interpretation: Second-degree heart block; Mobitz type II

Review Strip #34

Rate: 160
Rhythm: Regular
P wave: A
PRI: A
QRS: 0.24

Interpretation: Ventricular tachycardia

Review Strip #35

Rate: 80
Rhythm: Irregular
P wave: A
PRI: A
QRS: 0.12

Interpretation: Pacemaker rhythm (one beat failed to capture)

Review Strip #36

Rate: 70 (atrial)
Rhythm: Atrial rhythm: Regular
P wave: Present and upright
PRI: A
QRS: A

Interpretation: Ventricular standstill

Review Strip #37

Rate: 70
Rhythm: Regular
P wave: Present and upright
PRI: 0.16
QRS: 0.04

Interpretation: Normal sinus rhythm

Review Strip #38

Rate: 50
Rhythm: Regular
P wave: Present and upright
PRI: 0.20
QRS: 0.08

Interpretation: Sinus bradycardia

Review Strip #39

Rate: 20
Rhythm: Irregular
P wave: A
PRI: A
QRS: 0.20

Interpretation: Agonal rhythm

Review Strip #40

Rate: 90
Rhythm: Irregular
P wave: Present and upright (in normal complexes)
PRI: 0.16
QRS: 0.04

Interpretation: Sinus rhythm with a run of Ventricular Tachycardia (VT)

Review Strip #41

Rate: 80
Rhythm: Irregular
P wave: Present and upright (in normal complexes)
PRI: 0.06
QRS: 0.04

Interpretation: Sinus rhythm with multifocal couplet PVCs

Review Strip #42

Rate: 40
Rhythm: Irregular
P wave: Present and upright

PRI: Variable
QRS: Greater than 0.12

Interpretation: Third-degree heart block

Review Strip #43

Rate: 0
Rhythm: Irregular
P wave: A
PRI: A
QRS: A

Interpretation: Fine ventricular fibrillation

Review Strip #44

Rate: 90
Rhythm: Irregular
P wave: Present and upright
PRI: 0.12
QRS: 0.08

Interpretation: Sinus rhythm with unifocal PVCs

Review Strip #45

Rate: 60
Rhythm: Irregular
P wave: Present and upright
PRI: Progressively prolonging
QRS: 0.04

Interpretation: Mobitz type I; Wenchbach

Review Strip #46

Rate: 100
Rhythm: Irregular
P wave: I
PRI: A
QRS: 0.04

Interpretation: Atrial fibrillation

Review Strip #47

Rate: 70
Rhythm: Regular
P wave: Paced

PRI: 0.16
QRS: 0.04

Interpretation: Atrial pacemaker rhythm

Review Strip #48

Rate: 30
Rhythm: Regular
P wave: Present and upright
PRI: 0.16
QRS: 0.04

Interpretation: Sinus bradycardia

Review Strip #49

Rate: 130
Rhythm: Regular
P wave: A
PRI: A
QRS: Greater than 0.12

Interpretation: Ventricular tachycardia

Review Strip #50

Rate: Variable
Rhythm: Irregular
P wave: A
PRI: A
QRS: Greater than 0.12

Interpretation: Preshock, V fib; postshock, ventricular tachycardia

Review Strip #51

Rate: 70
Rhythm: Regular
P wave: Present and inverted
PRI: 0.14
QRS: 0.04

Interpretation: Accelerated junctional rhythm

Review Strip #52

Rate: 80
Rhythm: Regular

P wave: A
PRI: A
QRS: Greater than 0.12

Interpretation: Ventricular paced rhythm

Review Strip #53

Rate: 160
Rhythm: Irregular
P waves: A
PRI: A
QRS: I

Interpretation: Ventricular tachycardia

Review Strip #54

Rate: 70
Rhythm: Irregular
P wave: Present and upright
PRI: 0.20
QRS: 0.08

Interpretation: Sinus rhythm with frequent PVCs

Review Strip #55

Rate: 140
Rhythm: Regular
P wave: Present and upright
PRI: 0.18
QRS: 0.04

Interpretation: Sinus tachycardia

Review Strip #56

Rate: 110
Rhythm: Regular
P wave: Present and upright
PRI: 0.16
QRS: 0.08

Interpretation: Sinus tachycardia

Review Strip #57

Rate: 100
Rhythm: Regular

P wave: A
PRI: A
QRS: 0.12

Interpretation: Accelerated idioventricular rhythm

Review Strip #58

Rate: 90
Rhythm: Irregular
P wave: I
PRI: A
QRS: 0.08

Interpretation: Atrial fibrillation

Review Strip #59

Rate: 30
Rhythm: Irregular
P wave: A
PRI: A
QRS: Greater than 0.12

Interpretation: Agonal rhythm

Review Strip #60

Rate: 0
Rhythm: Irregular
P wave: A
PRI: A
QRS: A

Interpretation: Coarse ventricular tachycardia/ fibrillation

Review Strip #61

Rate: 70
Rhythm: Irregular
P wave: Present and upright
PRI: 0.16
QRS: 0.04

Interpretation: Sinus rhythm with a Premature Junctional Complex (PJC)

Review Strip #62

Rate: 70
Rhythm: Regular

P wave: Paced
PRI: 0.20
QRS: Greater than 0.12

Interpretation: AV sequential paced rhythm

Review Strip #63

Rate: 100
Rhythm: Irregular
P wave: Present, upright, and variable
PRI: 0.16
QRS: 0.04

Interpretation: Sinus dysrhythma

Review Strip #64

Rate: 40
Rhythm: Irregular
P wave: Present and upright
PRI: 0.24
QRS: 0.04

Interpretation: First-degree heart block with bi-geminy PVCs

Review Strip #65

Rate: 100
Rhythm: Regular
P wave: Present and upright
PRI: 0.24
QRS: 0.04

Interpretation: First-degree block

Review Strip #66

Rate: 60
Rhythm: Regular
P wave: Present and upright
PRI: 0.16
QRS: 0.04

Interpretation: Normal sinus rhythm

Review Strip #67

Rate: 50
Rhythm: Regular

P wave: Present and upright
PRI: 0.16
QRS: 0.04

Interpretation: Mobitz type II; second-degree heart block; 2:1 block

Review Strip #68

Rate: 90
Rhythm: Irregular
P wave: A
PRI: A
QRS: 0.12

Interpretation: Preshock, fine V fib; postshock, junctional rhythm

Review Strip #69

Rate: 70
Rhythm: Irregular
P wave: Present and upright
PRI: 0.16
QRS: 0.04

Interpretation: Sinus rhythm with a PVC

Review Strip #70

Rate: 30
Rhythm: Regular
P wave: Present and upright
PRI: 0.20
QRS: 0.04

Interpretation: Second-degree heart block; Mobitz type II; 3:1 block

Review Strip #71

Rate: 40
Rhythm: Irregular
P wave: Present and upright
PRI: Variable
QRS: 0.08

Interpretation: Third-degree block with a PAC

Review Strip #72

Rate: 20
Rhythm: Irregular
P wave: Present and upright
PRI: Variable
QRS: 0.12

Interpretation: Ventricular standstill with two idioventricular complexes

Review Strip #73

Rate: 30
Rhythm: Regular
P wave: Present and upright
PRI: Variable
QRS: 0.12

Interpretation: Third-degree heart block

Review Strip #74

Rate: 80
Rhythm: Irregular
P waves: Present and upright with normal
                 complexes
PRI: 0.16
QRS: 0.06

Interpretation: Sinus rhythm with PJCs

Review Strip #75

Rate: 40
Rhythm: Regular
P wave: 0
PRI: 0
QRS: Greater than 0.12

Interpretation: Idioventricular rhythm (IVR)

Review Strip #76

Rate: 180
Rhythm: Regular
P wave: Present and upright
PRI: 0.04
QRS: 0.04

Interpretation: Atrial tachycardia

Review Strip #77

Rate: 200
Rhythm: Irregular
P wave: 0
PRI: A
QRS: 0

Interpretation: Torsades de pointes

Review Strip #78

Rate: 80
Rhythm: Irregular
P wave: Present and upright
PRI: 0.16
QRS: 0.04

Interpretation: Sinus rhythm with PACs

Review Strip #79

Rate: 130
Rhythm: Irregular
P wave: Present and upright
PRI: 0.06
QRS: 0.04

Interpretation: Sinus tachycardia with PACs

Review Strip #80

Rate: 80
Rhythm: Regular
P wave: A
PRI: A
QRS: 0.04

Interpretation: Accelerated junctional tachycardia

Review Strip #81

Rate: 80
Rhythm: Irregular
P wave: Present and upright
PRI: 0.02
QRS: 0.04

Interpretation: Sinus dysrhythmia

Review Strip #82

Rate: 80
Rhythm: Irregular
P wave: Present and upright
PRI: 0.16
QRS: 0.04

Interpretation: Ventricular bigeminy

Review Strip #83

Rate: 80
Rhythm: Regular
P wave: Present and upright
PRI: 0.20
QRS: 0.04

Interpretation: Normal sinus rhythm with artifact

Review Strip #84

Rate: Ventricular rate, 20; atrial rate, 90
Rhythm: Atrial rhythm regular
P wave: Present and inverted
PRI: A
QRS: 0.12

Interpretation: Third-degree block

Review Strip #85

Rate: 80
Rhythm: Irregular
P wave: Present and upright
PRI: 0.16
QRS: 0.04

Interpretation: Sinus rhythm with couplet PVCs

Review Strip #86

Rate: 60
Rhythm: Irregular
P wave: Present and upright
PRI: Progressively prolonging
QRS: 0.04

Interpretation: Mobitz type I, second-degree block, Wechebach

Review Strip #87

Rate: Preshock, 200; postshock, 100
Rhythm: Preshock, irregular; postshock, irregular
P wave: I
PRI: A
QRS: Greater than 0.12 postshock

Interpretation: Preshock, coarse ventricular fibrillation; postshock, AIVR

Review Strip #88

Rate: 110
Rhythm: Irregular
P wave: Present and upright for normal complexes
PRI: 0.16
QRS: 0.08

Interpretation: Sinus tachycardia with 1 PVC and PJCs

Review Strip #89

Rate: 40
Rhythm: Regular
P wave: Present and upright
PRI: 0.20
QRS: 0.04

Interpretation: Sinus bradycardia

Review Strip #90

Rate: 150
Rhythm: Regular
P wave: Present and upright
PRI: 0.08
QRS: 0.04

Interpretation: Junctional tachycardia

Review Strip #91

Rate: 70
Rhythm: Irregular
P wave: Present and upright

PRI: 0.16
QRS: 0.04

Interpretation: Sinus rhythm with 2 PVCs

Review Strip #92

Rate: 180
Rhythm: Regular
P wave: Present and upright
PRI: 0.04
QRS: 0.04

Interpretation: Atrial tachycardia

Review Strip #93

Rate: 70
Rhythm: Regular
P wave: Present and inverted
PRI: 0.08
QRS: 0.04

Interpretation: Accelerated junctional rhythm

Review Strip #94

Rate: 100
Rhythm: Regular
P wave: A
PRI: A
QRS: 0.12

Interpretation: Ventricular tachycardia

Review Strip #95

Rate: 70
Rhythm: Regular
P wave: Present and upright
PRI: 0.28
QRS: 0.06

Interpretation: First-degree heart block

Review Strip #96

Rate: 40
Rhythm: Regular
P wave: Present and upright

PRI: Variable
QRS: 0.12

Interpretation: Third-degree block

Review Strip #97

Rate: 70
Rhythm: Irregular
P wave: Present and upright for normal complexes
PRI: 0.16
QRS: 0.04

Interpretation: Ventricular bigeminy

Review Strip #98

Rate: 40
Rhythm: Regular
P wave: Present and inverted
PRI: 0.08
QRS: 0.06

Interpretation: Junctional rhythm

Review Strip #99

Rate: 60
Rhythm: Regular
P wave: A
PRI: A
QRS: Greater than 0.12

Interpretation: Accelerated idioventricular rhythm

Review Strip #100

Rate: 70
Rhythm: Regular
P wave: Flutter waves
PRI: A
QRS: 0.04

Interpretation: Atrial flutter rhythm

Review Strip #101

Rate: 100
Rhythm: Regular

P wave: Present and upright
PRI: 0.16
QRS: 0.04

Interpretation: Normal sinus rhythm

Review Strip #102

Rate: Preshock, 200; postshock, 200
Rhythm: Preshock, irregular; postshock, irregular
P wave: I
PRI: A
QRS: Greater than 0.12 Preshock and postshock

Interpretation: Preshock, coarse ventricular fibrillation; postshock, coarse ventricular fibrillation

Review Strip #103

Rate: 20
Rhythm: Irregular
P Wave: A
PRI: A
QRS: Greater than 0.12

Interpretation: Idioventricular rhythm (agonal)

Review Strip #104

Rate: 80
Rhythm: Irregular
P wave: Present and upright
PRI: 0.14
QRS: 0.04

Interpretation: Normal sinus rhythm with unifocal PVC

Review Strip #105

Rate: 60
Rhythm: Regular
P wave: Present and upright (lot of artifact noted)
PRI: 0.12
QRS: 0.04

Interpretation: Normal sinus rhythm with artifact

Review Strip #106

Rate: 160
Rhythm: Regular
P wave: I
PRI: I
QRS: 0.10

Interpretation: Supraventricular tachycardia

Review Strip #107

Rate: 90
Rhythm: Regular
P wave: Present and upright
PRI: 0.16
QRS: 0.10

Interpretation: Normal sinus rhythm

Review Strip #108

Rate: 110
Rhythm: Regular
P wave: Present and upright
PRI: 0.16
QRS: 0.04

Interpretation: Sinus tachycardia with artifact at the first of the strip

Review Strip #109

Rate: 180
Rhythm: Irregular
P wave: I
PRI: A
QRS: 0.04

Interpretation: Atrial fibrillation with run of V tach and frequent unifocal PVCS

Review Strip #110

Rate: 120
Rhythm: Regular
P wave: Present and upright
PRI: 0.16
QRS: 0.04

Interpretation: Sinus tachycardia

Review Strip #111

Rate: 30
Rhythm: Irregular
P wave: I
PRI: A
QRS: 0.10

Interpretation: Atrial flutter

Review Strip #112

Rate: 70
Rhythm: Irregular
P wave: Present and upright
PRI: 0.12
QRS: 0.04

Interpretation: Sinus rhythm with PJC

Review Strip #113

Rate: 20
Rhythm: Irregular
P wave: I
PRI: A
QRS: Greater than 0.12

Interpretation: Idioventricular rhythm

Review Strip #114

Rate: Preshock, 200; postshock, 30
Rhythm: Preshock, irregular; postshock, irregular
P wave: I
PRI: A
QRS: Greater than 0.12 preshock and postshock

Interpretation: Preshock, coarse ventricular fibrillation; postshock, idioventricular rhythm

Review Strip #115

Rate: 120
Rhythm: Regular
P wave: Present and upright

PRI: 0.16
QRS: 0.08

Interpretation: Sinus tachycardia

Review Strip #116

Rate: 80
Rhythm: Irregular
P wave: Present and upright in normal
              complexes
PRI: 0.14 in normal complexes
QRS: 0.04 in normal complexes

Interpretation: Sinus rhythm with PJCs

Review Strip #117

Rate: 80
Rhythm: Regular
P wave: Present and upright
PRI: 0.16
QRS: 0.04

Interpretation: Normal sinus rhythm with inverted
T waves

Review Strip #118

Rate: 190
Rhythm: Regular
P wave: I
PRI: I
QRS: 0.04

Interpretation: Supraventricular tachycardia

Review Strip #119

Rate: 80
Rhythm: Regular
P wave: A
PRI: A
QRS: Greater than 0.12

Interpretation: AV sequential paced rhythm

Review Strip #120

Rate: 110
Rhythm: Irregular

P wave: A
PRI: A
QRS: 0.08

Interpretation: Accelerated junctional rhythm with
ventricular ectopic complexes

Review Strip #121

Rate: 90
Rhythm: Regular
P wave: Present and upright
PRI: 0.22
QRS: 0.08

Interpretation: Sinus rhythm with first-degree
block

Review Strip #122

Rate: 50
Rhythm: Regular
P wave: Present and upright (two per QRS)
PRI: 0.16
QRS: 0.04

Interpretation: Second-degree block Mobitz type
II, 2:1 block

Review Strip #123

Rate: 140
Rhythm: Regular
P wave: Present and upright
PRI: 0.16
QRS: 0.04

Interpretation: Sinus tachycardia

Review Strip #124

Rate: 30
Rhythm: Regular
P wave: Present and upright (three per QRS)
PRI: 0.16
QRS: 0.04

Interpretation: Second-degree block Mobitz type
II, 3:1 block

Review Strip #125

Rate: 50
Rhythm: Regular
P wave: Present and upright
PRI: Variable
QRS: 0.04

Interpretation: Third-degree block

Review Strip #126

Rate: 100
Rhythm: Irregular
P wave: I
PRI: I
QRS: 0.08

Interpretation: Atrial fibrillation

Review Strip #127

Rate: 170
Rhythm: Irregular
P wave: I
PRI: I
QRS: 0.06

Interpretation: Atrial fibrillation with rapid ventricular response

Review Strip #128

Rate: 80
Rhythm: Irregular
P wave: Present and upright
PRI: 0.12
QRS: 0.04

Interpretation: Sinus rhythm with PVC

Review Strip #129

Rate: 90
Rhythm: Regular
P wave: Present and upright
PRI: 0.20
QRS: 0.04

Interpretation: Normal sinus rhythm with ST segment elevation

Review Strip #130

Rate: 70
Rhythm: Irregular
P wave: Present and upright
PRI: 0.14
QRS: 0.04

Interpretation: Sinus rhythm with bigeminy PVC's

Review Strip #131

Rate: 30
Rhythm: Regular
P wave: A
PRI: A
QRS: 0.12

Interpretation: Idioventricular rhythm

Review Strip #132

Rate: 70
Rhythm: Irregular
P wave: Present and upright
PRI: 0.24
QRS: 0.04

Interpretation: Sinus rhythm with first-degree block and trigeminy PVCs

Review Strip #133

Rate: 80
Rhythm: Regular
P wave: Present and upright
PRI: 0.16
QRS: 0.04

Interpretation: Normal sinus rhythm with elevated ST segment

Review Strip #134

Rate: 111
Rhythm: Irregular
P wave: I
PRI: I
QRS: 0.08

Interpretation: Atrial fibrillation with rapid ventricular response

Review Strip #135

Rate:	70
Rhythm:	Irregular
P wave:	Present and upright
PRI:	0.16
QRS:	0.04

Interpretation: Normal sinus rhythm with PJCs

Review Strip #136

Rate:	60
Rhythm:	Irregular
P wave:	Present and upright
PRI:	0.20
QRS:	0.08

Interpretation: Normal sinus rhythm with PVCs

Review Strip #137

Rate:	130
Rhythm:	Regular
P wave:	I
PRI:	I
QRS:	0.06

Interpretation: Junctional tachycardia

Review Strip #138

Rate:	100
Rhythm:	Regular
P wave:	Present and upright
PRI:	0.12
QRS:	0.08

Interpretation: Normal sinus rhythm

Review Strip #139

Rate:	70
Rhythm:	Irregular
P wave:	Present and upright
PRI:	0.12
QRS:	0.04

Interpretation: Normal sinus rhythm with multi-focal PVCs

Review Strip #140

Rate:	60
Rhythm:	Regular
P wave:	Present and upright
PRI:	0.16
QRS:	0.08

Interpretation: Normal sinus rhythm

Review Strip #141

Rate:	40
Rhythm:	Regular
P wave:	Present and upright
PRI:	0.20
QRS:	0.04

Interpretation: Sinus bradycardia

Review Strip #142

Rate:	160
Rhythm:	Regular
P wave:	A
PRI:	A
QRS:	Greater than 0.12

Interpretation: Ventricular tachycardia

Review Strip #143

Rate:	50
Rhythm:	Irregular
P wave:	Present and upright
PRI:	0.20
QRS:	0.04

Interpretation: Sinus rhythm with PAC

Review Strip #144

Rate:	200+
Rhythm:	Irregular
P wave:	I
PRI:	I
QRS:	A

Interpretation: Ventricular fibrillation

Review Strip #145

Rate: 140
Rhythm: Regular
P wave: Present and upright
PRI: 0.16
QRS: 0.04

Interpretation: Sinus tachycardia

Review Strip #146

Rate: 80
Rhythm: Regular
P wave: Present and upright
PRI: 0.18
QRS: 0.06

Interpretation: Normal sinus rhythm

Review Strip #147

Rate: 50
Rhythm: Regular
P wave: Present and upright
PRI: 0.20
QRS: 0.04

Interpretation: Sinus bradycardia

Review Strip #148

Rate: 30
Rhythm: Irregular
P wave: Present and upright
PRI: I
QRS: 0.06

Interpretation: Third-degree block

Review Strip #149

Rate: 200+
Rhythm: Irregular
P wave: I
PRI: I
QRS: I

Interpretation: Ventricular fibrillation

Review Strip #150

Rate: 60
Rhythm: Regular
P wave: Present and upright
PRI: 0.28
QRS: 0.04

Interpretation: Normal sinus rhythm with first-degree block

Review Strip #151

Rate: 40
Rhythm: Regular
P wave: Present and upright
PRI: I
QRS: 0.08

Interpretation: Third-degree block

Review Strip #152

Rate: 50
Rhythm: Regular
P wave: Present and upright
PRI: 0.16
QRS: 0.04

Interpretation: Second-degree block Mobitz type II, 2:1 block

Review Strip #153

Rate: 200+
Rhythm: Irregular
P wave: I
PRI: I
QRS: I

Interpretation: Ventricular tachycardia turning into ventricular fibrillation

Review Strip #154

Rate: 30
Rhythm: Regular
P wave: A

PRI: A
QRS: Greater than 0.12

Interpretation: Idioventricular rhythm

Review Strip #155

Rate: 100
Rhythm: Regular
P wave: Present and upright
PRI: 0.20
QRS: 0.12

Interpretation: Normal sinus rhythm

Review Strip #156

Rate: 70
Rhythm: Regular
P wave: A
PRI: A
QRS: 0.08

Interpretation: Accelerated idioventricular rhythm

Review Strip #157

Rate: 80
Rhythm: Irregular
P wave: Present and upright
PRI: 0.12
QRS: 0.06

Interpretation: Sinus rhythm with premature atrial complex and inverted T wave

Review Strip #158

Rate: 80
Rhythm: Regular
P wave: Present and upright
PRI: 0.12
QRS: 0.04

Interpretation: Normal sinus rhythm

Review Strip #159

Rate: 200+
Rhythm: Irregular
P wave: A

PRI: A
QRS: I

Interpretation: Ventricular fibrillation

Review Strip #160

Rate: 70
Rhythm: Regular
P wave: Present and upright
PRI: 0.16
QRS: 0.04

Interpretation: Normal sinus rhythm

Review Strip #161

Rate: 100
Rhythm: Irregular
P Wave: Present and upright with normal complexes
PRI: 0.16
QRS: 0.04

Interpretation: Sinus rhythm with runs of V tach

Review Strip #162

Rate: 80
Rhythm: Regular
P wave: A
PRI: A
QRS: Greater than 0.12

Interpretation: Paced rhythm

Review Strip #163

Rate: 30
Rhythm: Regular
P wave: I
PRI: I
QRS: 0.04

Interpretation: Bradycardia, unable to determine sinus due to artifact

Review Strip #164

Rate: 100
Rhythm: Irregular

P wave: I
PRI: I
QRS: 0.04

Interpretation: Atrial fibrillation

Review Strip #165

Rate: 170
Rhythm: Irregular
P wave: I
PRI: I
QRS: 0.04

Interpretation: Supraventricular tachycardia with variable rate

Review Strip #166

Rate: 160
Rhythm: Irregular
P wave: I
PRI: I
QRS: 0.06

Interpretation: Atrial fibrillation with rapid ventricular response

Review Strip #167

Rate: 40
Rhythm: Regular
P wave: Present and upright
PRI: I
QRS: 0.04

Interpretation: Third-degree block

Review Strip #168

Rate: Preshock, 200; postshock, 60
Rhythm: Preshock, irregular; postshock, irregular
P wave: I
PRI: A
QRS: Greater than 0.12 pre- and postshock

Interpretation: Preshock, coarse ventricular fibrillation; postshock, idioventricular rhythm

Review Strip #169

Rate: 70
Rhythm: Regular
P wave: Present and upright
PRI: 0.14
QRS: 0.08

Interpretation: Normal sinus rhythm

Review Strip #170

Rate: 60
Rhythm: Regular
P wave: Present and upright
PRI: 0.20
QRS: 0.06

Interpretation: Normal sinus rhythm

Review Strip #171

Rate: 110
Rhythm: Regular
P wave: Present and upright
PRI: 0.12
QRS: 0.04

Interpretation: Sinus tachycardia

Review Strip #172

Rate: 40
Rhythm: Regular
P wave: A
PRI: A
QRS: 0.12

Interpretation: Idioventricular rhythm

Review Strip #173

Rate: 70
Rhythm: Regular
P Waves: Present and upright
PRI: 0.16
QRS: 0.04

Interpretation: Normal sinus rhythm

Review Strip #174

Rate: 90
Rhythm: Irregular
P wave: Present and upright
PRI: 0.22
QRS: 0.06

Interpretation: Sinus rhythm with first-degree block

Review Strip #175

Rate: 110
Rhythm: Regular
P wave: Present and upright
PRI: 0.16
QRS: 0.04

Interpretation: Sinus tachycardia

Review Strip #176

Rate: 40
Rhythm: Regular
P wave: Present and upright
PRI: V
QRS: 0.08

Interpretation: Third-degree block

Review Strip #177

Rate: 80
Rhythm: Regular
P wave: Present and upright
PRI: 0.12
QRS: 0.08

Interpretation: Wandering atrial pacer rhythm

Review Strip #178

Rate: 90
Rhythm: Irregular
P wave: Present and upright in normal complexes
PRI: 0.16
QRS: 0.06

Interpretation: Sinus rhythm with multifocal PVCs (bigeminy)

Review Strip #179

Rate: 200+
Rhythm: Irregular
P wave: A
PRI: A
QRS: A

Interpretation: Ventricular fibrillation

Review Strip #180

Rate: 110
Rhythm: Irregular
P wave: Present and upright
PRI: 0.12
QRS: 0.06

Interpretation: Sinus tachycardia with PJCs, PVC

Review Strip #181

Rate: 90
Rhythm: Regular
P wave: A
PRI: A
QRS: Greater than 0.12

Interpretation: Accelerated idioventricular rhythm

Review Strip #182

Rate: 60
Rhythm: Irregular
P Wave: A
PRI: A
QRS: I

Interpretation: Preshock, fine V fib; postshock, asystole

Review Strip #183

Rate: 120
Rhythm: Regular
P wave: A
PRI: A
QRS: Greater than 0.12

Interpretation: Ventricular tachycardia

Review Strip #184

Rate:	200
Rhythm:	Irregular
P wave:	A
PRI:	A
QRS:	I

Interpretation: Coarse V fib

Review Strip #185

Rate:	140
Rhythm:	Regular
P wave:	Present and upright
PRI:	0.16
QRS:	0.04

Interpretation: Sinus tachycardia

Review Strip #186

Rate:	90
Rhythm:	Regular
P wave:	A
PRI:	A
QRS:	0.04

Interpretation: Accelerated junctional rhythm

Review Strip #187

Rate:	70
Rhythm:	Regular
P wave:	F waves
PRI:	A
QRS:	0.04

Interpretation: Atrial flutter

Review Strip #188

Rate:	90
Rhythm:	Irregular
P wave:	f waves
PRI:	I
QRS:	0.06

Interpretation: Atrial fibrillation

Review Strip #189

Rate:	0
Rhythm:	0
P wave:	A
PRI:	A
QRS:	A

Interpretation: Asystole

Review Strip #190

Rate:	20
Rhythm:	Irregular
P wave:	Present and upright
PRI:	0.22
QRS:	0.06

Interpretation: First-degree block into asystole

Review Strip #191

Rate:	180
Rhythm:	Regular
P wave:	Present and upright
PRI:	0.12
QRS:	0.04

Interpretation: Supraventricular tachycardia

Review Strip #192

Rate:	40
Rhythm:	Regular
P wave:	Present and upright
PRI:	0.28
QRS:	0.06

Interpretation: Sinus bradycardia with first-degree heart block with ST segment elevation

Review Strip #193

Rate:	140
Rhythm:	Regular
P wave:	Present and upright
PRI:	0.16
QRS:	0.04

Interpretation: Sinus tachycardia

Review Strip #194

Rate: 60
Rhythm: Irregular
P wave: Present and upright
PRI: I
QRS: 0.10

Interpretation: Third-degree heart block with PVCs

Review Strip #195

Rate: 90
Rhythm: Irregular
P wave: Present and upright
PRI: 0.12
QRS: 0.06

Interpretation: Sinus rhythm with PJCs and PVCs

Review Strip #196

Rate: 20
Rhythm: Regular
P wave: Present and upright
PRI: 0.20
QRS: 0.08

Interpretation: Profound sinus bradycardia

Review Strip #197

Rate: 80
Rhythm: Regular
P wave: Present and upright
PRI: 0.18
QRS: 0.08

Interpretation: Normal sinus rhythm with ST segment elevation

Review Strip #198

Rate: 30
Rhythm: Regular
P wave: Present and upright
PRI: I
QRS: 0.06

Interpretation: Third-degree heart block

Review Strip #199

Rate: 50
Rhythm: Regular
P wave: Present and upright
PRI: 0.14
QRS: 0.04

Interpretation: Sinus bradycardia

Review Strip #200

Rate: 150
Rhythm: Irregular irregularity
P wave: I
PRI: I
QRS: 0.04

Interpretation: Atrial fibrillation runs of ventricular tachycardia

Review Strip #201

Rate: 140
Rhythm: Irregular irregularity
P wave: I
PRI: I
QRS: 0.04

Interpretation: Atrial fibrillation with rapid ventricular response, PVC

Review Strip #202

Rate: 70
Rhythm: Irregular
P wave: Present and upright
PRI: 0.16
QRS: 0.08

Interpretation: Sinus dysrhythmia rhythm with ST elevation

Review Strip #203

Rate: 70
Rhythm: Regular
P wave: A

PRI: A
QRS: 0.08

Interpretation: Accelerated junctional tachycardia

Review Strip #204

Rate: 20
Rhythm: Regular
P wave: Present and upright
PRI: A
QRS: Greater than 0.12

Interpretation: Third-degree heart block

Review Strip #205

Rate: 0
Rhythm: I
P wave: I
PRI: A
QRS: A

Interpretation: Asystole

Review Strip #206

Rate: 80
Rhythm: Regular
P wave: Present and upright
PRI: 0.16
QRS: 0.06

Interpretation: Sinus rhythm with ST segment depression (artifact)

Review Strip #207

Rate: 130
Rhythm: Irregular
P Wave: Present and upright
PRI: 0.18
QRS: 0.04

Interpretation: Sinus tachycardia with multifocal PVCs

Review Strip #208

Rate: 140
Rhythm: Regular

P wave: Present and upright
PRI: 0.16
QRS: 0.06

Interpretation: Sinus tachycardia

Review Strip #209

Rate: 70
Rhythm: Regular
P wave: Present and inverted
PRI: 0.08
QRS: 0.06

Interpretation: Accelerated junctional tachycardia

Review Strip #210

Rate: Greater than 200
Rhythm: Irregular
P wave: A
PRI: A
QRS: Variable

Interpretation: Torsades de pointes

Review Strip #211

Rate: 180
Rhythm: Regular
P wave: A
PRI: A
QRS: Greater than 0.12

Interpretation: Ventricular tachycardia

Review Strip #212

Rate: 220
Rhythm: Regular
P wave: I
PRI: I
QRS: 0.08

Interpretation: Supraventricular tachycardia

Review Strip #213

Rate: 90
Rhythm: Irregular
P wave: A

PRI: A
QRS: Greater than 0.12

Interpretation: Ventricular paced rhythm with occasional failure to capture

Review Strip #214

Rate: 30
Rhythm: Regular
P wave: Present and upright
PRI: Variable
QRS: 0.06

Interpretation: Third-degree heart block

Review Strip #215

Rate: 60
Rhythm: Regular
P Wave: Present and upright
PRI: 0.22
QRS: 0.06

Interpretation: Sinus rhythm with first-degree block

Review Strip #216

Rate: 40
Rhythm: Regular
P wave: Present and upright
PRI: 0.16
QRS: 0.06

Interpretation: Second-degree heart block, Mobitz type II

Review Strip #217

Rate: 60
Rhythm: Irregular
P wave: Present and upright
PRI: 0.16
QRS: 0.04

Interpretation: Sinus rhythm with PAC

Review Strip #218

Rate: 50
Rhythm: Irregular

P wave: Present and upright
PRI: 0.20
QRS: 0.06

Interpretation: Sinus bradycardia rhythm with a PVC

Review Strip #219

Rate: 90
Rhythm: Irregular irregularity
P wave: I
PRI: I
QRS: 0.04

Interpretation: Atrial fibrillation with multifocal and couplet PVCs

Review Strip #220

Rate: 90
Rhythm: Regular
P wave: Present and upright
PRI: 0.16
QRS: 0.06

Interpretation: Normal sinus rhythm

Review Strip #221

Rate: 70
Rhythm: Irregular
P wave: Present and upright
PRI: Variable
QRS: 0.06

Interpretation: Second-degree heart block, Mobitz type I

Review Strip #222

Rate: 70
Rhythm: Regular
P wave: A
PRI: A
QRS: Greater than 0.12

Interpretation: Sequential AV pacemaker rhythm

Review Strip #223

Rate:	70
Rhythm:	Regular
P wave:	Present and upright
PRI:	0.16
QRS:	0.04

Interpretation: Normal sinus rhythm

Review Strip #224

Rate:	80
Rhythm:	Regular
P wave:	Present and upright
PRI:	0.12
QRS:	0.04

Interpretation: Normal sinus rhythm

Review Strip #225

Rate:	80
Rhythm:	Irregular
P wave:	Present and upright
PRI:	0.12
QRS:	0.06

Interpretation: Sinus rhythm with bigeminy PVCs

Review Strip #226

Rate:	220
Rhythm:	Slightly irregular
P wave:	A
PRI:	A
QRS:	Greater than 0.12

Interpretation: Ventricular tachycardia

Review Strip #227

Rate:	112
Rhythm:	Regular
P wave:	Present and upright
PRI:	0.16
QRS:	0.08

Interpretation: Sinus tachycardia

Review Strip #228

Rate:	140
Rhythm:	Irregular irregularity
P wave:	I
PRI:	I
QRS:	0.06

Interpretation: Atrial fibrillation with rapid ventricular response

Review Strip #229

Rate:	70
Rhythm:	Regular
P wave:	A
PRI:	A
QRS:	Greater than 0.12

Interpretation: Ventricular paced rhythm

Review Strip #230

Rate:	100
Rhythm:	Regular
P wave:	Present and upright
PRI:	0.16
QRS:	0.04

Interpretation: Normal sinus rhythm

Review Strip #231

Rate:	90
Rhythm:	Irregular
P wave:	A
PRI:	A
QRS:	0.04

Interpretation: Atrial fibrillation with a PVC

Review Strip #232

Rate:	180
Rhythm:	Regular
P wave:	A
PRI:	A
QRS:	0.04

Interpretation: Supraventricular tachycardia

Review Strip #233

Rate: 70
Rhythm: Irregular
P wave: Present and upright
PRI: 0.16
QRS: 0.06

Interpretation: Normal sinus rhythm with unifocal PVCs

Review Strip #234

Rate: 60
Rhythm: Irregular
P wave: Present and upright
PRI: Variable
QRS: 0.08

Interpretation: Second-degree block type I with PVCs

Review Strip #235

Rate: 50
Rhythm: Regular
P wave: Present and upright
PRI: 0.20
QRS: 0.08

Interpretation: Sinus bradycardia

Review Strip #236

Rate: 90
Rhythm: Irregular
P wave: Present and upright
PRI: 0.12
QRS: 0.04

Interpretation: Sinus rhythm with PJCs

Review Strip #237

Rate: Preshock, Greater than 200; post-shock, 60
Rhythm: Preshock, irregular; postshock, regular
P wave: I
PRI: I
QRS: Preshock, I; postshock, 0.16

Interpretation: Preshock, V fib; postshock, IVR

Review Strip #238

Rate: 30
Rhythm: Regular
P wave: I
PRI: I
QRS: 0.10

Interpretation: Idioventricular rhythm

Review Strip #239

Rate: 60
Rhythm: Irregular
P wave: Present and upright
PRI: 0.18
QRS: 0.04

Interpretation: Sinus dysrhythmia rhythm

Review Strip #240

Rate: 80
Rhythm: Irregular
P wave: Present and upright
PRI: 0.16
QRS: 0.04

Interpretation: Sinus rhythm with unifocal PVCs

Review Strip #241

Rate: 50
Rhythm: Regular
P wave: A
PRI: A
QRS: 0.08

Interpretation: Junctional rhythm

Review Strip #242

Rate: 120
Rhythm: Regular
P wave: Present and upright
PRI: 0.16
QRS: 0.08

Interpretation: Sinus tachycardia

Review Strip #243

Rate: 70
Rhythm: Irregular
P wave: Present and upright
PRI: 0.16
QRS: 0.08

Interpretation: Sinus rhythm with PVCs

Review Strip #244

Rate: 180
Rhythm: Regular
P wave: A
PRI: A
QRS: Greater than 0.12

Interpretation: Ventricular tachycardia

Review Strip #245

Rate: 30
Rhythm: Regular
P wave: Present and upright
PRI: Variable
QRS: 0.06

Interpretation: Third-degree block

Review Strip #246

Rate: 100
Rhythm: Irregular
P wave: Present and upright
PRI: 0.18
QRS: 0.04

Interpretation: Sinus rhythm with bigeminy PVCs

Review Strip #247

Rate: 60
Rhythm: Regular
P wave: Present and upright
PRI: 0.22
QRS: 0.10

Interpretation: First-degree block

Review Strip #248

Rate: 90
Rhythm: Regular
P wave: A
PRI: A
QRS: Greater than 0.12

Interpretation: Ventricular pacemaker

Review Strip #249

Rate: 100
Rhythm: Irregular
P wave: Present and upright
PRI: 0.12
QRS: 0.04

Interpretation: Sinus rhythm with PJCs

Review Strip #250

Rate: 140
Rhythm: Irregular
P wave: I
PRI: I
QRS: 0.04

Interpretation: Atrial fibrillation, rapid ventricular response with multifocal PVCs

Review Strip #251

Rate: 30
Rhythm: Regular
P wave: A
PRI: A
QRS: 0.12

Interpretation: Idioventricular rhythm

Review Strip #252

Rate: 50
Rhythm: Irregular
P wave: Present and upright
PRI: Variable
QRS: 0.06

Interpretation: Third-degree heart block with multifocal PVCs

Review Strip #253

Rate: 110
Rhythm: Regular
P wave: Present and upright
PRI: 0.12
QRS: 0.08

Interpretation: Sinus tachycardia

Review Strip #254

Rate: 70
Rhythm: Irregular
P wave: Present and upright
PRI: 0.20
QRS: 0.06

Interpretation: Sinus rhythm; quadgeminy PVCs

Review Strip #255

Rate: 110
Rhythm: Irregular
P wave: Present and upright
PRI: 0.12
QRS: 0.04

Interpretation: Sinus tachycardia with sinus arrest

Review Strip #256

Rate: 0
Rhythm: 0
P wave: A
PRI: A
QRS: I

Interpretation: Coarse ventricular fibrillation

Review Strip #257

Rate: 50
Rhythm: Regular
P wave: Present and upright
PRI: 0.18
QRS: 0.04

Interpretation: Sinus bradycardia

Review Strip #258

Rate: 110
Rhythm: Irregular
P wave: Present and upright
PRI: 0.16
QRS: 0.04

Interpretation: Sinus rhythm with couplet PVCs

Review Strip #259

Rate: 70
Rhythm: Regular
P wave: Present and upright
PRI: 0.16
QRS: 0.10

Interpretation: Sinus rhythm

Review Strip #260

Rate: 180
Rhythm: Regular
P wave: A
PRI: A
QRS: 0.04

Interpretation: Supraventricular tachycardia

Review Strip #261

Rate: 40
Rhythm: Regular
P wave: A
PRI: A
QRS: Greater than 0.12

Interpretation: Idioventricular rhythm

Review Strip #262

Rate: 90
Rhythm: Irregular
P wave: F waves
PRI: I
QRS: 0.04

Interpretation: Atrial flutter with variable rate

Review Strip #263

Rate: 50
Rhythm: Regular
P wave: Inverted
PRI: 0.12
QRS: 0.08

Interpretation: Junctional rhythm

Review Strip #264

Rate: 60
Rhythm: Regular
P wave: Present and upright
PRI: 0.18
QRS: 0.04

Interpretation: Normal sinus rhythm with ST segment elevation

Review Strip #265

Rate: 50
Rhythm: Regular
P wave: Present and upright
PRI: 0.24
QRS: 0.04

Interpretation: Sinus bradycardia with first-degree block

Review Strip #266

Rate: 170
Rhythm: Regular
P wave: A
PRI: A
QRS: Greater than 0.12

Interpretation: Ventricular tachycardia

Review Strip #267

Rate: 50
Rhythm: Irregular
P wave: Present and upright
PRI: 0.14
QRS: 0.04

Interpretation: Sinus dysrhythmia

Review Strip #268

Rate: 110
Rhythm: Irregular
P wave: Present and upright
PRI: 0.12
QRS: 0.06

Interpretation: Sinus tachycardia with multifocal PVCs

Review Strip #269

Rate: 80
Rhythm: Regular
P wave: A
PRI: A
QRS: 0.06

Interpretation: Accelerated junctional rhythm

Review Strip #270

Rate: 70
Rhythm: Irregular
P wave: Present and upright
PRI: 0.16
QRS: 0.06

Interpretation: Wandering atrial pacemaker with a PVC

Review Strip #271

Rate: 130
Rhythm: Irregular
P wave: Present and upright
PRI: 0.16
QRS: 0.04

Interpretation: Sinus tachycardia with a PAC

Review Strip #272

Rate: 200
Rhythm: Irregular
P wave: A
PRI: A
QRS: 0.04

Interpretation: SVT into V tach

Review Strip #273

Rate: 30
Rhythm: Regular
P wave: Present and upright
PRI: Variable
QRS: 0.06

Interpretation: Third-degree heart block

Review Strip #274

Rate: Greater than 200
Rhythm: Irregular
P wave: A
PRI: A
QRS: Greater than 0.12 for ventricular complexes

Interpretation: Ventricular fibrillation with runs of V tach

Review Strip #275

Rate: 60
Rhythm: Regular
P wave: Present and upright
PRI: 0.20
QRS: 0.04

Interpretation: Sinus rhythm

Review Strip #276

Rate: 40
Rhythm: Regular
P wave: Present and upright
PRI: 0.20
QRS: 0.06

Interpretation: Sinus bradycardia with ST segment elevation

Review Strip #277

Rate: 90
Rhythm: Irregular
P wave: Present and upright
PRI: 0.12
QRS: 0.04

Interpretation: Sinus rhythm with PJCs

Review Strip #278

Rate: 70
Rhythm: Regular
P wave: A
PRI: A
QRS: 0.12

Interpretation: Ventricular paced rhythm

Review Strip #279

Rate: 140
Rhythm: Regular
P wave: Present and upright
PRI: 0.12
QRS: 0.04

Interpretation: Sinus tachycardia

Review Strip #280

Rate: 80
Rhythm: Irregular
P wave: Present and upright
PRI: 0.12
QRS: 0.08

Interpretation: Sinus rhythm with a PAC and a PVC

Review Strip #281

Rate: I
Rhythm: Irregular
P wave: A
PRI: A
QRS: 0.12 in discernible complexes

Interpretation: IVR going into ventricular fibrillation

Review Strip #282

Rate: 30
Rhythm: Regular

P wave: A
PRI: A
QRS: Greater than 0.12

Interpretation: Idioventricular rhythm

Review Strip #283

Rate: 50
Rhythm: Regular
P wave: Present and upright
PRI: Variable
QRS: 0.08

Interpretation: Third-degree block

Review Strip #284

Rate: 90
Rhythm: Irregular
P wave: Present and upright, biphasic
PRI: 0.16
QRS: 0.08

Interpretation: Sinus rhythm with a PAC

Review Strip #285

Rate: 190
Rhythm: Regular
P wave: A
PRI: A
QRS: 0.10

Interpretation: Ventricular tachycardia

Review Strip #286

Rate: 80
Rhythm: Regular
P wave: Present and upright
PRI: 0.16
QRS: 0.04

Interpretation: Normal sinus rhythm with depressed ST wave

Review Strip #287

Rate: 40
Rhythm: Irregular
P wave: Present and upright

PRI: Variable
QRS: 0.08

Interpretation: Third-degree block with PVCs

Review Strip #288

Rate: I
Rhythm: Irregular
P wave: A
PRI: A
QRS: I

Interpretation: Coarse V fib

Review Strip #289

Rate: 120
Rhythm: Regular
P wave: A
PRI: A
QRS: 0.08

Interpretation: Junctional tachycardia

Review Strip #290

Rate: 50
Rhythm: Regular
P wave: Present and upright
PRI: 0.22
QRS: 0.06

Interpretation: Sinus bradycardia with first-degree heart block, ST segment elevation

Review Strip #291

Rate: 140
Rhythm: Irregular
P wave: Present and upright in normal complexes
PRI: 0.16
QRS: 0.08

Interpretation: Sinus rhythm with run of V tach

Review Strip #292

Rate: 70
Rhythm: Regular

P wave: F waves
PRI: A
QRS: 0.08

Interpretation: Atrial flutter

Review Strip #293

Rate: 140
Rhythm: Regular
P wave: Present and upright
PRI: 0.12
QRS: 0.08

Interpretation: Sinus tachycardia

Review Strip #294

Rate: 180
Rhythm: Regular
P wave: A
PRI: A
QRS: 0.04

Interpretation: Supraventricular tachycardia

Review Strip #295

Rate: 30
Rhythm: Irregular
P wave: Present and upright
PRI: Variable
QRS: 0.06

Interpretation: Third-degree heart block with a PJC

Review Strip #296

Rate: 60
Rhythm: Regular
P wave: Present and upright
PRI: 0.18
QRS: 0.04

Interpretation: Sinus rhythm with ST segment elevation

Review Strip #297

Rate: 40
Rhythm: Regular

P wave: Present and upright
PRI: 0.16
QRS: 0.04

Interpretation: Second-degree heart block Type II; 2:1

Review Strip #298

Rate: I
Rhythm: Irregular
P wave: A
PRI: A
QRS: Greater than 0.12

Interpretation: Preshock, V tach; postshock, V fib

Review Strip #299

Rate: 60
Rhythm: Regular
P wave: Present and upright
PRI: 0.24
QRS: 0.06

Interpretation: First-degree heart block

Review Strip #300

Rate: 60
Rhythm: Regular
P wave: Present and upright
PRI: 0.20
QRS: 0.04

Interpretation: Normal sinus rhythm

Review Strip #301

Rate: 100
Rhythm: Irregular
P wave: Present and upright
PRI: 0.16
QRS: 0.08

Interpretation: Sinus rhythm with PJCs

Review Strip #302

Rate: 100
Rhythm: Irregular

P wave: Present and upright
PRI: 0.16
QRS: 0.08

Interpretation: Sinus rhythm with PVC

Review Strip #303

Rate: 140
Rhythm: Regular
P wave: Present and upright
PRI: 0.12
QRS: 0.04

Interpretation: Sinus tachycardia

Review Strip #304

Rate: 50
Rhythm: Irregular
P wave: Present and upright
PRI: 0.16
QRS: 0.10

Interpretation: Sinus bradycardia with PVCs

Review Strip #305

Rate: 60
Rhythm: Regular
P wave: Present and upright
PRI: 0.16
QRS: 0.04

Interpretation: Normal sinus rhythm with ST segment elevation

Review Strip #306

Rate: 80
Rhythm: Irregular
P wave: Present and upright
PRI: 0.12
QRS: 0.06

Interpretation: Normal sinus rhythm with PJC

Review Strip #307

Rate: 0
Rhythm: 0

P wave: A
PRI: A
QRS: A

Interpretation: Asystole

Review Strip #308

Rate: 100
Rhythm: Irregular
P wave: Present and upright
PRI: 0.16
QRS: 0.04

Interpretation: Normal sinus rhythm with PVC

Review Strip #309

Rate: 50
Rhythm: Regular
P wave: Present and upright (notched)
PRI: 0.16
QRS: 0.08

Interpretation: Sinus bradycardia

Review Strip #310

Rate: 80
Rhythm: Regular
P wave: A
PRI: A
QRS: 0.10

Interpretation: Accelerated junctional rhythm

Review Strip #311

Rate: Greater than 200
Rhythm: Irregular
P wave: I
PRI: I
QRS: I

Interpretation: Ventricular fibrillation

Review Strip #312

Rate: 100
Rhythm: Irregular

P wave: A (F waves)
PRI: A

Interpretation: Atrial flutter

Review Strip #313

Rate: 50
Rhythm: Regular
P wave: Present and upright
PRI: 0.16
QRS: 0.04

Interpretation: Sinus bradycardia

Review Strip #314

Rate: 60
Rhythm: Irregular
P wave: Present and upright
PRI: 0.22
QRS: 0.08

Interpretation: Sinus dysrhythmia with first-degree block

Review Strip #315

Rate: 70
Rhythm: Irregular
P wave: I
PRI: I
QRS: 0.08

Interpretation: Atrial fibrillation

Review Strip #316

Rate 30
Rhythm: Regular
P wave: A
PRI: A
QRS: 0.08

Interpretation: Junctional bradycardia

Review Strip #317

Rate: 70
Rhythm: Regular
P wave: Present and upright

PRI: 0.16
QRS: 0.08

Interpretation: Normal sinus rhythm with ST segment elevation

Review Strip #318

Rate: Greater than 200
Rhythm: Irregular
P wave: I
PRI: I
QRS: A

Interpretation: Ventricular fibrillation

Review Strip #319

Rate: 10
Rhythm: I
P wave: A
PRI: A
QRS: Greater than 0.12

Interpretation: Agonal rhythm

Review Strip #320

Rate: 60
Rhythm: Regular
P wave: Present and upright
PRI: 0.16
QRS: 0.04

Interpretation: Normal sinus rhythm

Review Strip #321

Rate: 100
Rhythm: Irregular
P wave: Present and upright
PRI: 0.16
QRS: 0.04

Interpretation: Sinus rhythm with PJCs

Review Strip #322

Rate: 140
Rhythm: Irregular
P wave: I

PRI: I
QRS: 0.04

Interpretation: Atrial fibrillation with rapid ventricular response

Review Strip #323

Rate: 40
Rhythm: Regular
P wave: Present and upright (notched)
PRI: 0.20
QRS: 0.08

Interpretation: Sinus bradycardia

Review Strip #324

Rate: 150
Rhythm: Regular
P wave: I
PRI: I
QRS: 0.04

Interpretation: Supraventricular tachycardia

Review Strip #325

Rate: 100
Rhythm: Regular
P wave: Present and upright
PRI: 0.16
QRS: 0.04

Interpretation: Normal sinus rhythm

Review Strip #326

Rate: Greater than 200
Rhythm: Irregular
P wave: I
PRI: I
QRS: I

Interpretation: Ventricular fibrillation

Review Strip #327

Rate: 50
Rhythm: Regular
P wave: Present and upright

PRI: 0.20
QRS: 0.04

Interpretation: Sinus bradycardia

Review Strip #328

Rate: 50
Rhythm: Irregular
P wave: Present and upright
PRI: 0.16
QRS: 0.04

Interpretation: Sinus bradycardia with PVC

Review Strip #329

Rate: 70
Rhythm: Irregular
P wave: Present and upright
PRI: 0.16
QRS: 0.4

Interpretation: Sinus dysrhythmia with ST segment elevation and a brief period (3 complexes) of first-degree block

Review Strip #330

Rate: 90
Rhythm: Irregular
P wave: Present and upright
PRI: 0.14
QRS: 0.04

Interpretation: Sinus rhythm with trigeminy PVCs

Review Strip #331

Rate: 110
Rhythm: Regular
P wave: Present and upright
PRI: 0.12
QRS: 0.04

Interpretation: Sinus tachycardia

Review Strip #332

Rate: 30
Rhythm: Regular
P wave: I

PRI: I
QRS: 0.08

Interpretation: Idioventricular rhythm

Review Strip #333

Rate: 150
Rhythm: Regular
P wave: Present and upright
PRI: 0.12
QRS: 0.08

Interpretation: Sinus tachycardia with artifact

Review Strip #334

Rate: 90
Rhythm: Irregular
P wave: Inverted (artifact also noted)
PRI: 0.12
QRS: 0.06

Interpretation: Junctional rhythm with multifocal PVC, bigeminy

Review Strip #335

Rate: Greater than 200
Rhythm: Irregular
P wave: I
PRI: I
QRS: I

Interpretation: Ventricular fibrillation

Review Strip #336

Rate: 40
Rhythm: Regular
P wave: Present and upright
PRI: 0.20
QRS: 0.06

Interpretation: Second-degree block, type II

Review Strip #337

Rate: 120
Rhythm: Regular
P wave: I

PRI: I
QRS: Greater than 0.12

Interpretation: Ventricular tachycardia

Review Strip #338

Rate: 80
Rhythm: Regular
P wave: Present and upright
PRI: 0.12
QRS: 0.08

Interpretation: Normal sinus rhythm with ST segment depression

Review Strip #339

Rate: 60
Rhythm: Regular
P wave: Present and upright
PRI: 0.20
QRS: 0.04

Interpretation: Normal sinus rhythm

Review Strip #340

Rate: 90
Rhythm: Irregular
P wave: A
PRI: A
QRS: 0.08

Interpretation: Junctional rhythm with bigeminy PVCs

Review Strip #341

Rate: 80
Rhythm: Regular
P wave: Present and upright
PRI: 0.12
QRS: 0.06

Interpretation: Normal sinus rhythm

Review Strip #342

Rate: 60
Rhythm: Regular

P wave: Present and upright
PRI: 0.22
QRS: 0.04

Interpretation: Sinus rhythm with first-degree block

Review Strip #343

Rate: 80
Rhythm: Regular
P wave: Present and upright
PRI: 0.20
QRS: 0.04

Interpretation: Normal sinus rhythm

Review Strip #344

Rate: 70
Rhythm: Irregular
P wave: A
PRI: A
QRS: 0.06

Interpretation: Junctional rhythm with bigeminy PVCs

Review Strip #345

Rate: 80
Rhythm: Regular
P wave: Present and upright
PRI: 0.16
QRS: 0.06

Interpretation: Normal sinus rhythm

Review Strip #346

Rate: 80
Rhythm: Irregular
P wave: Present and upright
PRI: 0.12
QRS: 0.04

Interpretation: Sinus rhythm with PJCs

Review Strip #347

Rate: 80
Rhythm: Regular

P wave: Present and upright
PRI: 0.12
QRS: 0.06

Interpretation: Normal sinus rhythm with ST segment elevation

Review Strip #348

Rate: 50
Rhythm: Regular
P wave: Present and upright (artifact also noted)
PRI: 0.22
QRS: 0.12

Interpretation: Sinus rhythm with first-degree block (with artifact)

Review Strip #349

Rate: Preshock, Greater than 200; post-shock, same
Rhythm: Preshock, irregular; postshock, irregular
P wave: Preshock, A; postshock, A
PRI: Preshock, A; postshock, A
QRS: Preshock, I; postshock, I

Interpretation: Ventricular fibrillation pre- and postshock

Review Strip #350

Rate: 30
Rhythm: Irregular
P wave: A
PRI: A
QRS: 0.10

Interpretation: Junctional bradycardia with PJC

Review Strip #351

Rate: 90
Rhythm: Irregular
P wave: Present and upright
PRI: 0.16
QRS: 0.06

Interpretation: Sinus rhythm with PAC and PVC

Review Strip #352

Rate: 50
Rhythm: Regular
P wave: Present and upright
PRI: 0.16
QRS: 0.04

Interpretation: Sinus bradycardia

Review Strip #353

Rate: 80
Rhythm: Irregular
P wave: I
PRI: I
QRS: 0.04

Interpretation: Atrial fibrillation with PVC

Review Strip #354

Rate: 80
Rhythm: Irregular
P wave: Present and upright
PRI: 0.16
QRS: 0.04

Interpretation: Marked sinus dysrhythmia

Review Strip #355

Rate: 60
Rhythm: Regular
P wave: Present and upright
PRI: 0.22
QRS: 0.10

Interpretation: Sinus rhythm with first-degree block

Review Strip #356

Rate: 180
Rhythm: Regular
P wave: I
PRI: I
QRS: 0.06

Interpretation: Supraventricular tachycardia

Review Strip #357

Rate: 30
Rhythm: Regular
P wave: A
PRI: A
QRS: 0.08

Interpretation: Idioventricular rhythm

Review Strip #358

Rate: 112
Rhythm: Irregular
P wave: Present and upright
PRI: 0.16
QRS: 0.04

Interpretation: Sinus rhythm with PVCs and run of PVCs

Review Strip #359

Rate: 60
Rhythm: Irregular
P wave: Present and upright
PRI: 0.20
QRS: 0.08

Interpretation: Sinus dysrhythmia with PVCs

Review Strip #360

Rate: Preshock, I; posstshock, 20
Rhythm: Preshock, irregular; postshock, regular
P wave: Preshock, A; postshock, A
PRI: Preshock, A; postshock, A
QRS: Preshock, I; postshock,0.12

Interpretation: Preshock, V fib; postshock, idioventricular rhythm

Review Strip #361

Rate: 50
Rhythm: Regular
P wave: Present and upright

PRI: 0.16
QRS: 0.06

Interpretation: Sinus bradycardia

Review Strip #362

Rate: 60
Rhythm: Irregular
P wave: A
PRI: A
QRS: 0.08

Interpretation: Junctional rhythm with PVC

Review Strip #363

Rate: Greater than 200
Rhythm: Irregular
P wave: A
PRI: A
QRS: I

Interpretation: Ventricular fibrillation pre- and postshock

Review Strip #364

Rate: 90
Rhythm: Irregular
P wave: I
PRI: I
QRS: 0.04

Interpretation: Atrial fibrillation with PVC

Review Strip #365

Rate: 80
Rhythm: Regular
P wave: A
PRI: A
QRS: 0.10

Interpretation: Accelerated junctional rhythm

Review Strip #366

Rate: 140
Rhythm: Regular

P wave: I
PRI: I
QRS: 0.08

Interpretation: Supraventricular tachycardia

Review Strip #367

Rate: 80
Rhythm: Irregular
P wave: I
PRI: I
QRS: 0.04

Interpretation: Atrial fibrillation with a PVC

Review Strip #368

Rate: 60
Rhythm: Regular
P wave: Present and upright (notched)
PRI: 0.20
QRS: 0.08

Interpretation: Normal sinus rhythm

Review Strip #369

Rate: 110
Rhythm: Regular
P wave: Present and upright
PRI: 0.20
QRS: 0.04

Interpretation: Sinus tachycardia

Review Strip #370

Rate: 80
Rhythm: Regular
P wave: Present and upright
PRI: 0.12
QRS: 0.04

Interpretation: Normal sinus rhythm

Review Strip #371

Rate: 100
Rhythm: Irregular

P wave: Present and upright
PRI: 0.20
QRS: 0.06

Interpretation: Sinus rhythm with bigeminy PVCs

Review Strip #372

Rate: 50
Rhythm: Irregular
P wave: Present and upright
PRI: Variable
QRS: 0.10

Interpretation: Third-degree block with PVCs

Review Strip #373

Rate: 30
Rhythm: Regular
P wave: A
PRI: A
QRS: 0.08

Interpretation: Idioventricular rhythm

Review Strip #374

Rate: 80
Rhythm: Irregular
P wave: I
PRI: I
QRS: 0.04

Interpretation: Atrial fibrillation

Review Strip #375

Rate: 80
Rhythm: Regular
P wave: A
PRI: A
QRS: 0.10

Interpretation: Accelerated idioventricular rhythm

Review Strip #376

Rate: 80
Rhythm: Regular

P wave: Present and upright
PRI: 0.24
QRS: 0.06

Interpretation: Sinus rhythm with first-degree block with ST segment elevation

Review Strip #377

Rate: 50
Rhythm: Regular
P wave: A
PRI: A
QRS: 0.04

Interpretation: Junctional rhythm

Review Strip #378

Rate: 60
Rhythm: Irregular
P wave: Present and upright
PRI: 0.16
QRS: 0.10

Interpretation: Sinus rhythm with PVC and ST segment elevation

Review Strip #379

Rate: 200
Rhythm: Regular
P wave: A
PRI: A
QRS: 0.12

Interpretation: Supraventricular tachycardia changing to ventricular tachycardia

Review Strip #380

Rate: Preshock, 200; postshock, 0
Rhythm: Preshock, regular; postshock, A
P wave: Preshock, A; postshock, A
PRI: Preshock, A; postshock, A
QRS: Preshock, 0.12; postshock, A

Interpretation: Preshock, V tach; postshock, ventricular standstill

Review Strip #381

Rate: 60
Rhythm: Irregular
P wave: A
PRI: A
QRS: 0.04

Interpretation: Atrial fibrillation

Review Strip #382

Rate: 120
Rhythm: Regular
P wave: Present and upright
PRI: 0.12
QRS: 0.04

Interpretation: Sinus tachycardia

Review Strip #383

Rate: 80
Rhythm: Regular
P wave: Present and upright
PRI: 0.20
QRS: 0.04

Interpretation: Normal sinus rhythm

Review Strip #384

Rate: 200
Rhythm: Regular
P wave: A
PRI: A
QRS: 0.04

Interpretation: Supraventricular tachycardia

Review Strip #385

Rate: 70
Rhythm: Regular
P wave: Present and upright
PRI: 0.20
QRS: 0.06

Interpretation: Sinus dysrhythmia

Review Strip #386

Rate: 80
Rhythm: Regular
P wave: Present and upright
PRI: 0.22
QRS: 0.04

Interpretation: Sinus rhythm with first-degree block

Review Strip #387

Rate: Preshock, 200; postshock, 0
Rhythm: Preshock, irregular; postshock, A
P wave: Preshock, A; postshock, A
PRI: Preshock, A; postshock, A
QRS: Preshock, I; postshock, A

Interpretation: Preshock, V fib; postshock, asystole

Review Strip #388

Rate: 70
Rhythm: Irregular
P wave: Present and upright
PRI: 0.16
QRS: 0.04

Interpretation: Sinus rhythm with PVC

Review Strip #389

Rate: 40
Rhythm: Regular
P wave: A
PRI: A
QRS: 0.06

Interpretation: Junctional rhythm

Review Strip #390

Rate: 120
Rhythm: Regular
P wave: A
PRI: A
QRS: Greater than 0.12

Interpretation: Ventricular tachycardia

Review Strip #391

Rate: 90
Rhythm: Regular
P wave: A
PRI: A
QRS: 0.04

Interpretation: Accelerated junctional rhythm

Review Strip #392

Rate: 80
Rhythm: Irregular
P wave: Present and upright
PRI: 0.12
QRS: 0.04

Interpretation: Sinus rhythm with quadrigeminy PVCs

Review Strip #393

Rate: 80
Rhythm: Irregular
P wave: I due to artifact
PRI: I due to artifact
QRS: 0.04

Interpretation: Sinus rhythm with PVC (artifact)

Review Strip #394

Rate: 0
Rhythm: 0
P wave: 0
PRI: 0
QRS: 0

Interpretation: Asystole

Review Strip #395

Rate: Greater than 200
Rhythm: Irregular
P wave: A
PRI: A
QRS: Greater than 0.12

Interpretation: Torsades de pointes

Review Strip #396

Rate: 70
Rhythm: Regular
P wave: Present and upright
PRI: 0.22
QRS: 0.04

Interpretation: Sinus rhythm with first-degree block

Review Strip #397

Rate: 120
Rhythm: Regular
P wave: Present and upright
PRI: 0.12
QRS: 0.04

Interpretation: Sinus tachycardia

Review Strip #398

Rate: 20
Rhythm: Irregular
P wave: Present and upright
PRI: 0.16
QRS: 0.04

Interpretation: Profound sinus bradycardia with atrial standstill

Review Strip #399

Rate: 70
Rhythm: Irregular
P wave: Present and upright
PRI: 0.16
QRS: 0.04

Interpretation: Sinus rhythm with bigeminy PVCs with a couplet of PVCs

Review Strip #400

Rate: 30
Rhythm: Regular
P wave: A
PRI: A
QRS: Greater than 0.12

Interpretation: Idioventricular rhythm

Index